# Immunology
## A Laboratory Manual
### Second Edition

# Immunology
## A Laboratory Manual
### Second Edition

Richard L. Myers
*Southwest Missouri State University*

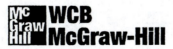

WCB
McGraw-Hill

Boston   Burr Ridge, IL   Dubuque, IA   Madison, WI   New York   San Francisco   St. Louis
Bangkok   Bogotá   Caracas   Lisbon   London   Madrid
Mexico City   Milan   New Delhi   Seoul   Singapore   Sydney   Taipei   Toronto

# McGraw-Hill Higher Education

*A Division of The McGraw·Hill Companies*

**Book Team**

Editor  *Elizabeth M. Sievers*
Production Editor  *Kay Driscoll*
Photo Editor  *Carrie Burger*
Art Processor  *Renee Grevas/Joyce Watters*

Vice President and General Manager  *Beverly Kolz*
Vice President, Publisher  *Kevin Kane*
Vice President, Director of Sales and Marketing  *Virginia S. Moffat*
Vice President, Director of Production  *Colleen A. Yonda*
National Sales Manager  *Douglas J. DiNardo*
Marketing Manager  *Patrick E. Reidy*
Advertising Manager  *Janelle Keeffer*
Production Editorial Manager  *Renée Menne*
Publishing Services Manager  *Karen J. Slaght*
Royalty/Permissions Manager  *Connie Allendorf*

President and Chief Executive Officer  *G. Franklin Lewis*
Senior Vice President, Operations  *James H. Higby*
Corporate Senior Vice President, President of WCB Manufacturing  *Roger Meyer*
Corporate Senior Vice President and Chief Financial Officer  *Robert Chesterman*

Copyedited by Pam Humbert

Cover/interior design by Lesiak/Crampton Design, Inc.
Cover images © Photo Researchers

Library of Congress Catalog Card Number: 94–71467

ISBN 0–697–11313–2

Printed in the United States of America by Wm. C. Brown Communications, Inc.,
2460 Kerper Boulevard, Dubuque, IA 52001

10  9  8  7

# Contents

# *Preface*

As a student studying immunology, I grew increasingly fascinated by immunology laboratory exercises that answered so many questions about theoretical concepts of immunobiology. No other area of biology offered such a clear and obvious approach to scientific questions. It included all the basics of scientific exploration: a bounty of questions, a base of information upon which to plan an experimental strategy, and methods to use to obtain the desired information. Now, as a teacher and researcher, I continue to be interested and amazed and find my students equally excited about the methodology of immunology. While the techniques have become more sophisticated, they still apply to student inquisition.

This laboratory manual seeks to bring together a group of methods that provides an experimental foundation for the beginning immunology student. The manual, intended for the student enrolled in a beginning course that has a laboratory component, supplements current textbooks. Many instructors use the first exercise—the preparation and use of a vaccine—to initiate a course because the exercise contains a variety of learning components.

The student then explores a series of procedures that serves as an introduction to immunology from both the **applied** and **experimental** viewpoints. Topics for these exercises represent current areas of study that provide a significant amount of the clinical and research information reported in today's important journals. All of the exercises are simple enough that beginning students can follow and appreciate them, but complex enough to produce meaningful results.

The manual is divided into five sections. An introduction to basic immunology laboratory techniques is followed by a section dealing with immunoassays. The next section deals with antibody detection, isolation and analysis. The fourth section stresses cell techniques and provides the base necessary to comprehend advanced techniques. The final section includes a group of procedures not necessarily related to each other but selected because of their contemporary importance.

Although each exercise can be performed without completion of previous exercises, each relates to the proceeding exercises. This develops student laboratory prowess and maturity in immunology. Exercises were chosen and designed with the realization that a student has limited time to spend in the laboratory. With some preparation, a student can complete at least half of these exercises within a two-hour period. Other exercises take more time and require the student (and instructor) to plan and manage time wisely. The introduction to each section provides a graph relating the amount of **instructor preparation time** and **student time** necessary to successfully complete each exercise. This is intended to be only a guide for the instructor and student and necessarily relies upon a thorough understanding of the procedures.

The manual provides more exercises than most students can complete in one semester, so the instructor can choose those deemed most relevant and appropriate. Some exercises may not be appropriate for some institutions because of restrictions for use of radioisotopes. Although most of the exercises do not require sophisticated and expensive equipment, some do require instrumentation (e.g., scintillation counter). Enough exercises are included, however, to allow the instructor to choose those that best meet the course requirements and facility limitations.

I hope that this manual will provide direction and perhaps inspiration for young and aspiring immunologists. My wife, Kathy, and daughters, Barbra and Ashley, have been inspirational and patient during the preparation of this book. I thank them for their support. I am also indebted to Janice Horton for her expert advice and technical assistance.

# *Introductory Immunology Procedures*

The first section of this laboratory manual acquaints the beginning immunology student with some fundamental principles of **laboratory immunobiology.** These four exercises use a variety of basic techniques to develop sound laboratory skills that will be important in subsequent sections.

The first exercise, an intricate, long-term project, deals with the **preparation and use of a vaccine** followed by an assessment of the efficiency of the vaccine. It may require an entire semester to complete. Some instructors may ask students to complete exercise 2 and perhaps others before beginning exercise 1, because these exercises introduce concepts that may be helpful for successful completion of exercise 1. Students will find exercise 1 useful in learning to **design experiments** and **schedule experimentation.** Collaborative study and work are encouraged and perhaps necessary for successful completion. The exercise includes an introduction to the care and use of **laboratory animals** and stresses student obligations when performing animal research.

The immunizing agents chosen represent different classes of antigens, and each choice requires mastery of unique techniques. For example, microbiological and aseptic techniques become particularly important to students using a pathogenic bacterium as an immunizing agent. Finally, this exercise provides the base for ambitious students to continue independent study under the supervision of the instructor. This exercise, along with exercises presented in section III, may be used by the instructor as the basis for a term paper which may be written in the style of a research paper submitted for publication. The antiserum prepared in exercise 1 can be analyzed by procedures in section III. The author has found that other students in the class serve as excellent reviewers for the submitted paper.

The second exercise reviews **dilution procedures** and stresses practice and refinement of pipetting skills. It also builds confidence in the student's laboratory abilities by strengthening manipulative skills. The first segment emphasizes the meaning of **dilution** and **titer.** A colored substance is diluted and the effect of dilution visibly interpreted. Secondly, red blood cells are exposed to a detergent which lyses them. The results of exposure to increasing dilutions of the detergent reinforce the idea that dilution moderates the effects of an active substance. This exercise also serves as an introduction to serology.

Exercise 3 is devoted entirely to the **study of blood.** Although it stresses the composition of whole blood, the exercise deals primarily with the separation of cells and emphasizes the study of the cellular elements of blood. It provides the background required by several following exercises. Routine white cell counts and differential cell counts will be performed to aid student identification and handling of the formed elements of blood.

The final exercise, presented for comparative purposes, stresses the importance of **natural resistance** to disease. It examines the filtering capacity of the mammalian circulatory system and auxiliary lymphoid organs. In a related experiment, murine phagocytic cells are fed bacterial cells in vitro and, after non-phagocytized bacteria are removed, macrophages are observed microscopically. Bacteria either adhering to the macrophage or internalized will be visible, emphasizing the important role of this cell in natural resistance.

*Figure I presents the approximate instructor preparation time and student laboratory time necessary for successful completion of exercises 1 through 4.*

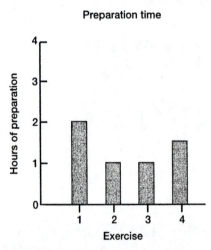
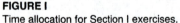
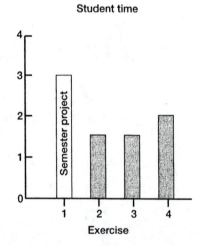

**FIGURE I**
Time allocation for Section I exercises.

# Vaccination—A Semester Project

## INTRODUCTION

This exercise introduces the student to the procedures involved in the: (1) preparation of a vaccine, (2) appropriate use of the vaccine; and (3) determination of the efficiency of the vaccine. As a result of this work, the student will understand **immunization procedures** that result in antibody synthesis and also develop an awareness of the basis for the immune response. Students may use the exercise as a foundation for procedures that follow.

## MATERIALS

(Per pair)

A. Bacterial vaccine

    4 plates of brain heart infusion agar (BHIA)

    1 24-hr culture of attenuated *Salmonella typhi* (or other species)

    1 bottle of sterile saline

    1 sterile screw-cap tube

    2 sterile tubes

    2 tubes brain heart infusion broth (BHIB)

    3 sterile vaccine bottles

    1 hemacytometer and coverslip

    1 12-ml syringe with 18-gauge needle

    1-, 5- and 10-ml pipettes

    Anaerobic jar

    Water bath (100° C)

    Gram stain materials

    Crystal Violet

B. Erythrocyte vaccine

    2 sterile graduated centrifuge tubes

    3 sterile vaccine bottles

    2 tubes brain heart infusion broth (BHIB)

    1 12-ml syringe with 18-gauge needle

    2 20-ml syringes with 22-gauge needles

    1 bottle sterile saline

    Heparin

    Tourniquet

    Alcohol swabs

    Adhesive bandages

    Sterile capillary pipettes

    10-ml pipettes

    Anaerobic jar

C. Protein vaccine

    1 bottle sterile saline

    2 tubes brain heart infusion broth (BHIB)

    3 sterile vaccine bottles

    1 12-ml syringe and 18-gauge needle

    Egg albumin (or other protein)

    1% thimerosal (merthiolate) or filter-sterilization apparatus

    Anaerobic jar

D. Other techniques

    1. Injections

        1 tuberculin syringe and needle

        Alcohol swabs

        Razor or single-edge razor blade

        Soap

        Restraining box

    2. Bleeding the rabbit

        1 50-ml syringe and 18-gauge needle

        70% ethanol

        Restraining table

        Ketamine hydrochloride (Sigma, St. Louis, MO)

        Balance (for rabbit weight)

    3. Preparation of serum

        1 100-ml sterile screw-cap bottle

        Sterile capillary pipette

        Sterile vaccine bottle

        Sterile centrifuge tubes

## PROCEDURE

### Preparation of a Vaccine

Many biological molecules and cells can elicit an immune response. One result of the stimulation of the **immune response** is the stimulation of certain lymphoid cells by anti-

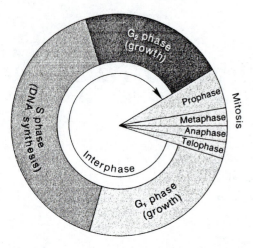

**FIGURE 1.1**

The life cycle of a lymphocyte. Once activated by antigen, B cells differentiate into blast cells that begin antibody synthesis. Blast cells will differentiate further into either antibody-secreting plasma cells or memory cells.

From Stuart Ira Fox, *Human Physiology*, 2d ed. Copyright © 1987 Wm. C. Brown Publishers, Dubuque, Iowa. All Rights Reserved. Reprinted by permission.

gen followed by the production of antibody. Antibody production occurs during the latter stages of the G1 phase and the early stages of the S phase of the cell life cycle (figure 1.1).

In this exercise students will choose a substance to be used as a vaccine. Selection depends upon the desired result (e.g., protection from a bacterial infection). Students may choose from: (a) bacteria, (b) erythrocytes, (c) soluble proteins, or (d) other antigens selected by the instructor. However, each student should understand the procedures involved in the other vaccine preparations.

### Bacterial Vaccine

Bacteria, a composite of **antigenic determinants** (epitopes), elicit the formation of a variety of antibodies. Many of these antibodies produce excellent in vitro reactions and these reactions can be used to quantitate the efficiency of the bacterial vaccine. Bacterial vaccines, sometimes called *bacterins,* are suspensions of bacteria that have been inactivated so that disease is not produced but yet antigenicity is retained. Figure 1.2 shows a typical response to a bacterial vaccine.

To produce a bacterial vaccine, one must: (1) culture bacteria, (2) wash and dilute the bacteria appropriately, and (3) inactivate and preserve them. The following procedure is designed to produce a vaccine to be used to immunize an animal to *Salmonella typhi,* the cause of typhoid fever. Other bacterial species may be used depending upon the discretion of the instructor.

1.  Inoculate the surface of plates of brain heart infusion agar (BHIA) with *Salmonella typhi* so that maximum growth occurs on the agar surface. Incubate the plates at 37° C for 18 to 24 hr.

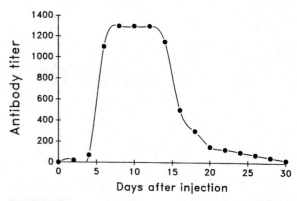

**FIGURE 1.2**

A typical immune response to a bacterial vaccine. A rabbit was injected with $5 \times 10^8$ bacteria on day 0, and its serum was assayed for antibody titer for a period of 30 days.

**Assume this microorganism to be pathogenic and use appropriate aseptic techniques.**

2.  After incubation, pipette approximately 2 ml of sterile saline onto the surface of the plates and loosen the growth with a sterile inoculating loop. Pipette the bacterial suspension into a sterile tube. **Do not mouth pipette.** Mix to obtain a suspension of cells free of clumps.

3.  Gram stain the cells to determine the purity of the culture.

4.  Place the bacterial cells in a sterile screw-cap tube and heat in a 100° C water bath for 1 hr. This should kill the cells without adversely affecting the antigenicity of the somatic or "O" antigens. The **killed cells** will serve as the vaccine. Distinguish between "O" and "H" antigens on this microorganism.

5.  Check for complete killing (sterilization) by inoculating 2 tubes of prereduced, sterile brain heart infusion broth (BHIB) or other appropriate media with vaccine. Incubate one anaerobically and the other aerobically at 37° C for 48 hr. In the meantime, store the vaccine in a vaccine bottle at 4° C until sterility is verified. Growth in BHIB indicates improper sterilization (or contamination), and the vaccine cannot be used.

6.  Centrifuge the killed, suspended cells at $1,500 \times g$ for 10 min and discard the supernatant. Add 10 ml of sterile saline and mix to obtain an even suspension of killed bacteria.

7.  Prepare a series of ten-fold dilutions from a portion of the cell suspension to obtain the appropriate dilution to determine the number of bacteria per ml of original suspension using a hemacytometer. A drop of crystal violet added to an appropriate dilution (probably 1:1,000) will make the cells easier to see. Follow the procedure for use of a hemacytometer outlined on page 5.

8. After determining the number of bacteria in the killed suspension, dilute to $5 \times 10^9$ bacteria per ml in saline.
9. Dispense the diluted bacteria into a sterile, sealed and labelled vaccine bottle with a sterile needle and syringe and store at 4° C until needed.

### Use of the Hemacytometer

1. Place a clean microscope coverslip over the counting chamber of a hemacytometer. Do not cover the grooved area so that a sample of cells can be applied to the groove with a sterile capillary pipette.
2. Apply a drop of the stained cell suspension (begin with the 1:1,000 dilution) and allow the cells to run under the coverslip and fill the counting chamber. Let the cells settle for a few minutes before counting.
3. Using the high-dry objective of the microscope, count the cells in 80 of the smallest squares. An adjustment of the condenser and iris diaphragm may help to make cells more visible. It is best to count blocks of 16 of the smallest squares, the 4 blocks at the corners and the one in the middle of the grid, designated 1 through 5 in figure 1.3. Only cells within the squares and those touching the edges should be counted.
4. To determine the number of bacteria per ml of the original suspension using the number of cells counted with the hemacytometer, see the explanation in the appendix.
5. The hemacytometer method will be used in later exercises to determine the number of white blood cells as well as the number of bacteria in suspension.

### Erythrocyte Vaccine

Erythrocytes (red blood cells) also make excellent antigens. These, like bacteria, contain many antigenic determinant sites and elicit a good immune response in appropriate experimental animals. For example, specific epitopes form the basis for typing blood. The procedure for the preparation of erythrocytes for injection involves (1) aseptic collection of blood, (2) addition of an anticlotting agent, and (3) cell washing and dilution.

1. Collect approximately 5 ml of blood in a syringe containing heparin (0.1 mg/ml). Blood may be taken from a human volunteer by a **trained phlebotomist** under the supervision of the instructor. Many phlebotomists prefer to use the Becton Dickinson Vacutainer® system for blood collection. Alternatively, blood may be taken from an experimental animal other than that

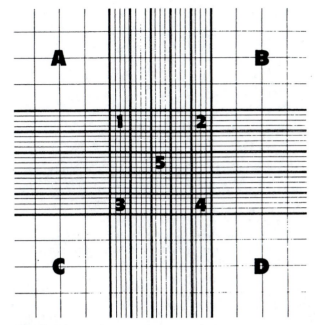

**FIGURE 1.3**
The hemacytometer grid. The 80 small squares in sections 1–5 are used for red blood cell and bacterial cell counts. The larger squares in sections A, B, C and D are used for white blood cell counts.
From Stuart Ira Fox, *Human Physiology*, 2d ed. Copyright © 1987 Wm. C. Brown Publishers, Dubuque, Iowa. All Rights Reserved. Reprinted by permission.

chosen for vaccination. Always follow safety procedures outlined by the instructor, which includes the proper use and disposal of needles.
2. Place the heparinized blood in a sterile centrifuge tube and centrifuge at $1,500 \times g$ for 5 min. Aspirate the fluid portion (plasma) with a sterile capillary pipette and discard.
3. Wash the cells 3 times in sterile physiological saline and discard the saline after each wash. Centrifuge at $1,500 \times g$ for 5 min each wash.
4. Make a 25% suspension of the washed cells in saline. Use the graduations on the centrifuge tube for this procedure and **mix carefully** until the red cells are suspended. Dispense into sterile, sealed vaccine bottles. Remember that **erythrocytes are fragile.** Aspirating or dispensing with too much pressure will cause lysis.
5. Check for contamination by inoculating 2 tubes of prereduced BHIB or other appropriate media and incubating one anaerobically and the other aerobically at 37° C for 48 hr. Store the labelled erythrocyte vaccine at 4° C until sterility is assured or until needed. Erythrocyte vaccines have a limited storage life. After a few weeks of storage, students will have to discard the vaccine and repeat the preparation. Any bacterial growth indicates contamination, and the vaccine, if contaminated, **should not be used.**

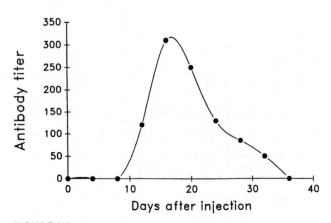

**FIGURE 1.4**
A typical immune response to a protein vaccine. A rabbit was injected with horse serum on day 0, and its serum was assayed for antibody titer for a period of 36 days.

## Protein Vaccine

Many soluble proteins that are derived from animals are antigenic. These have varying capacities to elicit an immune response, and, therefore, the choice of protein must be made carefully in order to achieve a measurable response such as that shown in figure 1.4. Soluble proteins such as serum albumin, gamma globulin, or egg albumin make excellent choices. Egg albumin (ovalbumin) is suggested for this exercise.

1.  Prepare a 1% solution of egg albumin by weighing out 0.5 g of crystalline egg albumin and adding 49.5 ml of sterile saline. Place the mixture in a cold room and wait for the protein to go into solution before proceeding. **Do not stir.** Stirring will produce foam, which may cause problems.
2.  Sterilization may be achieved by adding thimerosal to a final concentration of 1:5,000, or the solution may be filter-sterilized using a 0.45 μ membrane filter attached to a 50 ml syringe. More than one filter may have to be used to successfully filter the entire volume.
3.  Check for sterility of the preparation by inoculating 2 tubes of prereduced BHIB or other appropriate media with the vaccine and incubating one anaerobically and the other aerobically at 37° C for 48 hr.
4.  Dispense into sterile, sealed and labelled vaccine bottles and store at 4° C until needed. **Do not use** the vaccine if bacterial growth is present.

## Use of the Vaccine

### The Use of Experimental Animals

Without the use of experimental animals, knowledge of the biological sciences would not be at the advanced stage enjoyed today. Experimental animals have provided model systems for the exploration of basic principles that have hastened our understanding of phenomena associated with all life processes. Use of experimental animals is a privilege which **should not be taken for granted.** Strict regulations govern the use of animals in biological laboratories to ensure the humane treatment and use of this valuable resource. Regulations should be closely followed and use monitored by a special committee. The care and use of animals will be discussed in detail by your instructor. Make certain that you understand all rules and regulations before proceeding.

The instructor should demonstrate the injection and bleeding of animals before any work is attempted. Rabbits will be used, and each pair of students will be assigned an individual rabbit. Your instructor may decide to use rats or mice for this experiment. Although students will work in pairs, each student is responsible for the proper **use and care** of the experimental animal. Follow the instructor's directions carefully. To properly inject and bleed, the student must handle the animal firmly but carefully to prevent undue harm to the animal or the student.

### Injections

Material can be injected through a number of routes, including (1) subcutaneous, (2) intraperitoneal, (3) intravenous, and sometimes (4) intracardial. Inoculations require the use of a sterile needle and syringe, and the size of each depends upon the route of injections and the volume to be delivered. Needles are categorized according to gauge (smaller numbers represent larger needles) and length. Syringes are categorized as to volume. A commonly used needle and syringe is the tuberculin syringe which is a 1-ml syringe with a 26 or 27 gauge, ½ inch needle. Table 1.1 provides additional information about the sizes of needles used for injection. This table lists the appropriate needle gauge for injection of rabbits. All of the procedures that follow apply to all species and will be referenced in later exercises.

1.  *Subcutaneous Injection*
    a.  This method involves the injection of material under the skin. Choose a site (usually the back for convenience), clip and shave the hair, and disinfect the injection site with 70% ethanol.

**Table 1.1**  Different Injection Routes Require Different Needle Sizes

| Injection Route | Needle Gauge |
| --- | --- |
| Cardiac puncture | 18 |
| Intraperitoneal | 20 to 24 |
| Subcutaneous | 23 to 26 |
| Intravenous | 25 to 27 |

b. Load a tuberculin syringe and insert the needle almost horizontal to the animal to a depth of approximately ⅛ in.

c. Slowly inject the inoculum and observe the formation of a slightly raised area (bleb) under the skin.

d. Remove the needle and disinfect the injection site once again with alcohol.

2. *Intraperitoneal Injection*

a. Using this procedure the student will inject material into the peritoneal or abdominal cavity of the animal. An assistant's help will be necessary, or, alternatively, the rabbit should be immobilized on a board especially built to restrain the animal on its back. Anesthesia may be used for this injection. (See "Bleeding the rabbit" below.)

b. Clip the hair away from the injection site and disinfect the site with 70% ethanol. Grasp the skin and peritoneum with the fingers and insert the needle through the skin and peritoneum.

c. Inject the inoculum carefully so as to prevent injection into abdominal organs. With practice the procedure is relatively easy.

d. Remove the needle and disinfect the area once again with alcohol.

3. *Intravenous Injection*

a. This procedure involves direct injection into the bloodstream of the animal. The marginal ear vein is the most accessible and visible vein in the rabbit and, therefore, is most commonly used. The student will see the vein clearly on the dorsal edge of either ear. Specially designed rabbit boxes are available to restrain the rabbit so that intravenous injection is simplified (see figure 1.5).

b. Shave the hair away from the area with a razor or a single-edge razor blade. Cleanse the area and disinfect it with 70% ethanol.

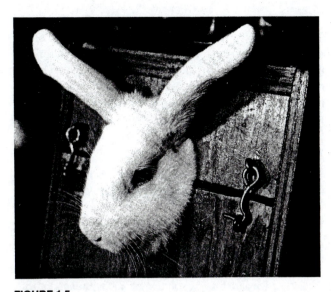

**FIGURE 1.5**
A rabbit box designed to hold the rabbit's head motionless so that injections can be made into the marginal ear vein.

c. For ease of injection, the diameter of the vein may be enlarged before injection by trauma (rubbing, thumping, heating) and by applying pressure over the vein at the base of the ear.

d. Hold the ear with one hand while supporting the ear from below with fingers of the same hand.

e. With the vein clearly visible, insert the needle in the direction of the blood flow (towards the head of the rabbit). Slowly inject the inoculum while watching for signs of dilution of blood in the vein indicating that the injected material is passing into the vein. The plunger of the syringe should move down easily and no raised area in the surrounding tissue should be visible.

f. If the vein is missed, try again to inject into the same vein but a few centimeters toward the head of the animal. When the injection is complete, withdraw the needle and administer firm pressure with the fingers to the injection site to stop bleeding.

g. Disinfect the area with alcohol.

### Bleeding the Rabbit

Bleeding from the heart, commonly called cardiac puncture, is often used to obtain hyperimmune serum from the rabbit after the vaccination procedure is complete. Your instructor, however, may choose to have students obtain blood for antibody titration from the marginal ear vein. Be sure to listen carefully to instructions.

To the beginning student the cardiac puncture appears to be the most difficult procedure in this exercise. However, with a thorough explanation by the instructor and practice and patience by the student, it will prove to be the most rapid and successful method for obtaining a sufficient amount of serum for in vitro antibody titration. If the procedure is carried out as described, the rabbit will not be harmed and, in fact, may be bled a number of times whenever serum is desired.

1. Cardiac bleeding is best done when the rabbit is securely tied to a specially designed restraining table and anesthetized. The animal must remain motionless during the entire procedure, and success depends upon careful preparation.
2. Anesthetize the rabbit with ketamine hydrochloride, a short-term surgical anesthesia. Prepare a stock solution of 200 mg/ml and inject 0.15 ml/lb of body weight intramuscularly. This should provide ample time to perform the cardiac bleeding. Note: Always monitor vital signs before, during, and after anesthesia.
3. Many technicians prefer to clip the hair from the thorax to a few centimeters below the sternum. This gives a better view of the area so that the needle can be inserted into the area of the heart with confidence. Apply 70% ethanol to the clipped area.
4. Attach an 18-gauge needle to a suitable syringe and free the plunger. By gently touching the rabbit around the area on the left side of the midline with your finger, you will feel a slight heartbeat. With a firm grip on the syringe, insert the needle between the ribs while pulling the plunger. As the insertion is made, it is possible to feel the pulsation of the heart as the needle touches it. Continue to insert the needle and watch for blood to flow into the syringe. At this point, stop advancing the needle and hold the syringe steady until the desired amount of blood has been drawn. As much as 50 ml of blood may be taken from a large rabbit without adverse effects.
5. Withdraw the needle slowly. Often the student misses the heart on the first attempt, so the needle should be withdrawn slowly and once again advanced. Many instructors prefer to bleed the rabbit by inserting the needle just to the left of the xiphoid cartilage at the base of the sternum.

*Preparation of Serum*

Whole blood is composed of cellular and fluid portions. Serum is the clear, straw-colored liquid that results after clotting is complete. This exercise requires serum. Since clotting is desired, no anticoagulants are used when the blood is collected. After collection, the student must quickly dispense the blood into sterile, clean glassware. The serum that is seen after clotting is complete will contain the antibodies that will be quantified. The quantity of antibody produced depends upon the efficiency of the vaccine.

1. Dispense the blood into 100-ml, sterile, clean, screw-cap bottles immediately after collection. Place in a 4° C cold room. Blood may be left in the cold room overnight.
2. After completing the clotting process, withdraw the serum with a sterile capillary pipette and dispense it into sterile, sealed vaccine bottles. Discard the clot.
3. If the serum is not perfectly clear, centrifuge it in sterile, clean centrifuge tubes at $1,800 \times g$ for 10 min. Collect the serum and discard the cells.

*Immunization Schedules*

Experimental animals do not respond equally to all vaccines. For consistent results, however, use care in the preparation and administration of the vaccine. Since results vary from animal to animal, some alterations in the injection schedule may produce better results.

Trial bleedings may be done periodically to determine the rabbit's immunological response. Blood needed for this may be taken from the marginal ear vein since only a small volume is necessary.

Protein vaccines **may produce anaphylaxis** (why?) and the student will want to watch for symptoms of anaphylaxis during the last few protein injections. In addition, carefully monitor the animals during this entire exercise for any symptoms of poor health (in which case the instructor should be notified and appropriate action taken).

All vaccine injections should be done intravenously. Table 1.2 provides protocols that produce adequate results. Bacteria should be prepared at a suspension of $5 \times 10^9$ cells/ml; erythrocytes at a 25% suspension; protein at a 1% solution.

**Table 1.2** Suggested Injection Schedules for Bacterial, Erythrocyte and Protein Vaccines

| Inject on Day: | Bacteria (ml) | Erythrocytes (ml) | Protein (ml) |
|---|---|---|---|
| 1 | 0.1 | 1.0 | 0.1 |
| 2 | — | 1.0 | — |
| 3 | 0.25 | 1.0 | 0.5 |
| 4 | — | — | — |
| 5 | 0.25 | 1.0 | 1.0 |
| 6 | — | — | — |
| 7 | — | 1.0 | 1.0 |
| 8 | 0.5 | — | — |
| 9 | — | — | 1.0 |
| 10 | 0.75 | 1.0 | — |
| 11 | — | — | — |
| 12 | 1.0 | — | 1.0 |

## Determination of the Efficiency of the Vaccine

Each antiserum will be assayed for antibody by a procedure that will be presented in later exercises and completed by the class prior to the time when it will be needed for this exercise. **Titer,** the term used to describe the antibody concentration, is usually expressed as the reciprocal of the highest dilution that gives a visible antigen-antibody reaction. Antisera to bacteria and erythrocytes will be titered using an **agglutination reaction.** Antisera to egg albumin will be assayed by a **precipitation reaction.**

## DISCUSSION

Vaccination has had a significant impact on health. However, certain problems are inherent in vaccine production. An example is the liberation of endotoxin due to lysis when Gram-negative bacteria are autoclaved. Autoclaving, therefore, could certainly not be used in the preparation of a vaccine from Gram-negative bacteria.

Students must adhere to strict schedules to make exercise 1 successful. This necessarily requires extra (unscheduled) time in the laboratory. Because students work in pairs, each student must accept certain responsibilities and, when unable to meet schedules, let others know so that the success of the exercise is not jeopardized.

*Salmonella typhi* is a pathogen and certainly poses problems for individuals not acquainted with aseptic technique and handling of infectious microorganisms. Substitutions may be made at the discretion of the instructor. Most human *Salmonella* pathogens are found in species I

(cholerae-suis). This leaves a large number from which to select since more than 2,000 different serovars of *Salmonella* exist.

As discussed, the cardiac puncture is the most expeditious method for obtaining blood for serological purposes. The student may, however, decide to bleed the rabbit from the ear to avoid possible trauma. Alternatively, the instructor may assign rats or mice for this experiment instead of rabbits.

Comparisons of titers of vaccines can be made, but other types of comparisons are meaningless. Some students may want to determine if cross-reactions exist. For example, serum raised to *S. typhi* could be tested to determine if it agglutinates sheep red blood cells. A more significant experiment would be a comparison of anti-*S. typhi* cross-reactivity with closely related species or genera.

## SELECTED REFERENCES

Flecknell, P. A., 1984. The relief of pain in laboratory animals. *Lab. Anim.* 18:147.

Germanier, R., ed. 1985. *Bacterial vaccines.* Orlando, FL: Academic Press, Inc.

Green, C. J. 1978. Anesthesia and analgesia. In *Laboratory animals: An introduction for new experimenters,* edited by A. A. Tuffery, pp. 261–301. Chichester, England: John Wiley and Sons.

*Guide for the care and use of laboratory animals.* 1985. U.S. Department of Health and Human Services. Public Health Services. National Institutes of Health. NIH Publication No. 85:23.

Harkness, J. E., and J. E. Wagner. 1989. *The biology and medicine of rabbits and rodents.* 3d edition. Philadelphia, PA: Lea and Febiger.

John, P. C. L., ed. 1981. *The cell cycle.* Cambridge, England: Cambridge University Press.

Lerner, R. A. 1983. Synthetic vaccines. *Sci. Am.* 248:66.

McLaughlin, C. A., and R. B. Chiasson. 1979. *Laboratory anatomy of the rabbit.* 2d edition. Dubuque, IA: Wm. C. Brown.

Mitchison, N. A. 1984. Rational design of vaccines. *Nature.* 308:112.

*Public health service policy on humane care and use of laboratory animals.* 1986. Bethesda, MD: Office for Protection from Research Risks, National Institutes of Health.

Wilson, I. A., H. L. Norman, R. A. Houghton, et al. 1984. The structure of an antigenic determinant in a protein. *Cell.* 37:767.

EXERCISE

# 2

# *The Dilution Concept*

## INTRODUCTION

This exercise illustrates the meaning of **dilution** or **titration.** The methods presented here are used in many immunological and serological procedures where it is necessary to determine the activity or content of a reagent or serum. For example, the dilution of serum determines antibody content for diagnostic purposes. The procedures and associated skills demonstrated in this exercise also play an important role in the later exercises.

These techniques provide only estimates of actual content. Exercise caution in performing the procedures, especially pipetting, so that the limited accuracy obtained is not sacrificed. These procedures will produce results that are good enough to use to make conclusions about the content of the material in question.

All dilution procedures utilize a **diluent** (solution) that will not adversely affect material such as antibodies, other biological molecules, or cells being diluted. One popular diluent is physiological saline, an aqueous solution of 0.85% sodium chloride. Often this is buffered at pH 7 to pH 7.4 with phosphate and is appropriately called **phosphate buffered saline** (PBS). The salt is at a physiological concentration, and the pH is compatible with mammalian cells and systems. One may choose from many other solutions such as Ringer solution that provide the desired results, but keep in mind that the results of the dilution should not be altered because of reactions between the diluent and material diluted.

A routine dilution procedure involves the serial (successive) dilution of antigen or antibody. Commonly, two-fold dilutions are made such as 1:2, 1:4, 1:8, 1:16, etc. Ten-fold dilutions are also useful and result in dilutions of 1:10 ($10^{-1}$), 1:100 ($10^{-2}$), 1:1,000 ($10^{-3}$), 1:10,000 ($10^{-4}$), etc. Both dilution procedures contain relatively large experimental error; use other techniques when a more quantitative measure is desired.

For the two-fold dilution scheme place a constant volume of diluent (e.g., 0.5 or 1.0 ml) in a series of tubes. An equal volume of the material to be diluted is placed in the first tube and thoroughly mixed. The same volume is then transferred to the next tube. This procedure is repeated through the last tube (figure 2.1). The excess volume from the last tube is discarded, other reactants are added, and the tubes are carefully examined for visible endpoint reaction.

Immunologic endpoints may be precipitation, agglutination, flocculation, hemagglutination, etc., and represent the hypothetical concentration of reactant in the non-diluted material. The endpoint is referred to as the *titer.* The titer is expressed as the **reciprocal of the highest dilution** that shows the endpoint.

The reaction temperature is important and perhaps critical. Immunological and serological reactions may occur over a wide range of temperatures, usually determined by the nature of the material studied in the titration. The most useful temperature, however, is 37° C, and most clinical and research dilutions and titrations are performed at this temperature. Constant temperature water baths provide the critical temperature, because substances heat uniformly in water baths.

For accurate and reproducible results the student must correctly use serological pipettes. Most pipettes are manufactured to precise specifications and, when used properly, deliver the appropriate amount. Your laboratory instructor will demonstrate the use of pipettes.

In addition to practice with dilution schemes, the following procedures demonstrate: (1) a ten-fold dilution of a colored dye that produces a visible endpoint, and (2) a two-fold dilution of a detergent that lyses erythrocytes (figure 2.2).

## MATERIALS

(Per pair)

> 0.85% saline
>
> 1 tube 0.5% sodium dodecyl sulfate in saline (other hemolyzing solutions such as Triton X-100 or Steron SE may be used)
>
> 1 tube 2% sheep erythrocytes (SRBC)
>
> Serological tubes (10 × 75- and 16 × 150-mm)
>
> Tube holders
>
> 1- and 10-ml pipettes
>
> Water bath (37° C)
>
> Capillary pipettes
>
> Methylene blue dye solution (1% aqueous solution)
>
> Vortex mixer
>
> Distilled water
>
> Centrifuge

**11**

## PROCEDURE

### Tenfold Dilutions

In this part of the exercise, the student will use a ten-fold dilution scheme to dilute a colored dye to the point where no color remains. This is analogous to the dilution of serum proteins or other biological substances. Eventually, so few dye molecules remain that the unaided eye perceives no color. Likewise, antibody can be diluted to the point where there are not sufficient antibodies to produce a visible reaction. This scheme is useful when the substance being titrated has a high activity. It is, of course, subject to error, and good technique is extremely important. It is good practice to use a different pipette with each transfer. For more precise determinations of titer, one would prepare another series of more critical dilutions on either side of the endpoint.

1. Set up a series of 5, 16 × 150-mm tubes in a rack. A 1:10 ($10^{-1}$), 1:100 ($10^{-2}$), 1:1,000 ($10^{-3}$), 1:10,000 ($10^{-4}$) and 1:100,000 ($10^{-5}$) dilution should be prepared. Label the tubes appropriately.
2. Use a 10-ml pipette to add 9.0 ml of water to each of the 5 tubes. Your instructor may have you use an **autopipette** or a **micropipette** to obtain the same result in this and other exercises that require small volumes. Pay particular attention to the use of the pipette in this step and steps to follow. Skills mastered at this point will be important in later exercises.
3. With a 1-ml pipette, transfer 1 ml of the methylene blue dye solution into the first tube ($10^{-1}$). Mix with a vortex mixer. Mixing, a critical step in dilution procedures, must be done properly to ensure transfer of a representative sample to the next tube. Notice the intensity of the blue color.
4. Transfer 1 ml from the $10^{-1}$ tube into the second tube ($10^{-2}$). Mix and once again notice the color intensity. Does the color appear to be less intense?
5. Continue this procedure through the last tube. One ml may be discarded from the last tube to maintain a constant volume in all tubes.
6. Finally, **visually** compare all 5 tubes. The color intensity should diminish as the methylene blue is sequentially diluted. Each tube represents a dilution that is 10 times greater than the previous one.

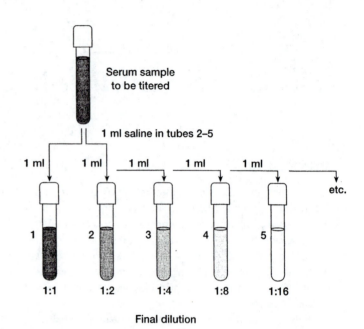

**FIGURE 2.1**
A diagram of a two-fold dilution scheme. Dilutions are important in many immunological procedures. Careful use of the pipette is necessary for accurate results.

### Twofold Dilutions

Erythrocytes or red blood cells (RBC) are fragile and may lyse in hypotonic saline solutions. Many materials such as solvents, surface active agents, and microbial toxins, as well as antibodies, have the capacity to lyse RBC. When lysis occurs, hemoglobin, a red conjugated protein, is liberated. Each hemoglobin molecule consists of one globin molecule and four heme molecules; the heme is responsible for the color of the entire compound. In this exercise the detergent, sodium dodecyl sulfate (SDS), will be used to demonstrate lysis of RBC. The student will see that SDS may be diluted to the point that lysis no longer occurs. A two-fold dilution scheme will be used.

1. Prepare a series of ten serological tubes (10 × 75 mm) in a rack. Make certain that the tubes are **thoroughly cleaned** so that false reactions will not occur because of lysis by contaminating chemicals. Number the tubes.
2. Carefully pipette 1.0 ml of physiological saline into tubes 2 through 10 with a 1 ml serological pipette. As before, autopipettes or micropipettes may be used to obtain the desired results.

3. Carefully pipette 1.0 ml of 0.5% SDS in saline into tubes 1 and 2. Tube 1 represents the **control tube** (undiluted control).

4. Mix the contents of tube 2 and carefully pipette 1.0 ml from tube 2 into tube 3. Mix. With a clean pipette transfer 1.0 ml from tube 3 into tube 4. Repeat the procedure through tube 9. Discard 1.0 ml from tube 9. Tube 10 will serve as the saline control (no lysis). Each tube should now contain 1.0 ml.

5. Add 1.0 ml of a 2% SRBC suspension to each of the 10 tubes. *Carefully* mix the contents of each tube. Make certain that the SRBC are not mechanically lysed.

6. Incubate all tubes in a 37° C water bath for 15 min.

7. Observe the hemolysis. Erythrocytes not lysed will settle to the bottom of the tube within 2 hr, and the pellet size will represent the degree of hemolysis. Hemolysis may also be determined by the red color (wine color) of the supernatant. The intensity of the red indicates the degree of hemolysis. To speed up the experiment, the tubes may be centrifuged (500 × g for 10 min) after incubation to pellet intact red cells.

8. Record the titer as the last tube (highest dilution of reagent) that has obvious hemolysis.

## DISCUSSION

Projects involving dilutions present particular problems for many students. These can be overcome by working through hypothetical dilution problems using dilution schemes and flowsheets such as that presented in figure 2.1. The technique of pipetting must also be mastered before reproducible results can be expected. Experienced technicians use micropipetters that can deliver volumes of 10 μl or less without error for routine serial deliveries in the immunology laboratory.

Erythrocytes (and other cells) are particularly susceptible to lysis by many chemicals. Biological molecules are also destroyed by certain chemicals. These chemicals may be contaminants on glassware; therefore, glassware that is not absolutely clean creates misleading results. Special glassware detergents that remove blood, fats, soil, etc., without leaving a residue should be used for critical cleaning. Many clinicians and researchers use disposable glassware or plasticware to avoid the problem of dirty materials.

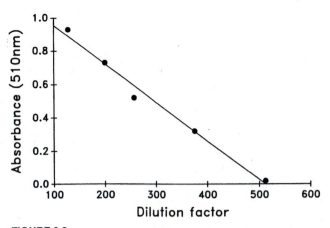

**FIGURE 2.2**
The results obtained when the detergent, SDS, is serially diluted and added to a suspension of erythrocytes. As the detergent is diluted, lysis of erythrocytes is reduced.

## SELECTED REFERENCES

Peacock, J. E., and R. H. Tomar. 1980. *Manual of laboratory immunology.* Philadelphia, PA: Lea and Febiger.

Rose, N. R., E. C. de Macario, J. L. Fahey, H. Friedman, and G. M. Penn, eds. 1992. *Manual of clinical laboratory immunology.* 4th ed. Washington, DC: American Society for Microbiology.

# 3

# *The Study of Blood*

## INTRODUCTION

This exercise provides a background in **hematology.** The procedures presented will be useful for successful completion of further exercises.

Blood is a fluid which contains cellular elements and a number of molecules necessary to feed the tissues and regulate functions of the body. The fluid and cellular elements that are shown in figure 3.1 can be easily separated by centrifugation. The cellular elements can be stationary within tissue or circulate with the blood itself. The fluid portion contains an aqueous solution of salts, carbohydrates, and proteins.

Blood is of interest to the immunologist (and serologist). Most immune mechanisms have their origin in specific blood cells, and the fluid portion contains molecules that regulate and are the products of the immune system.

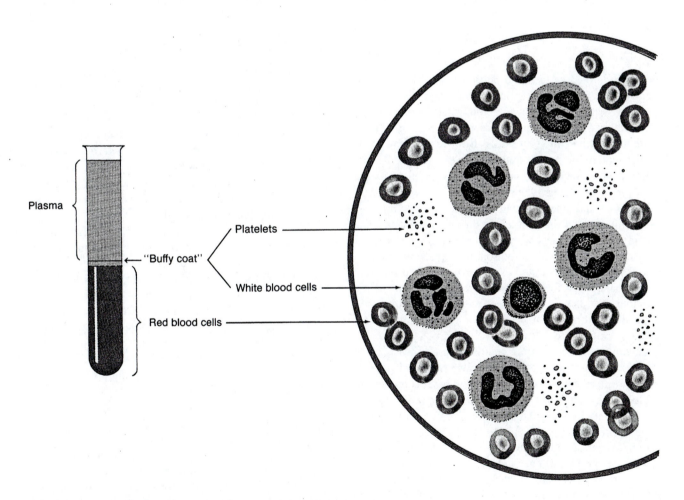

Plasma

"Buffy coat"

Platelets

White blood cells

Red blood cells

**FIGURE 3.1**
Blood cells become packed at the bottom of the tube when whole blood is centrifuged, leaving the fluid plasma at the top of the tube. Red blood cells (erythrocytes) are the most abundant of the blood cells. White blood cells (leukocytes) and platelets form only a thin, light-colored "buffy coat" at the interface between the packed red blood cells and the plasma.

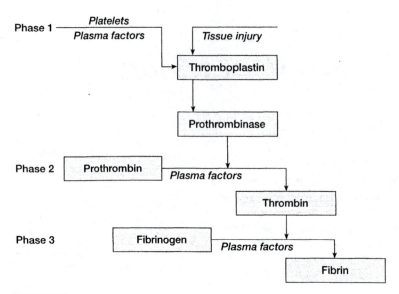

**FIGURE 3.2**
The mechanism of blood clotting. This pathway leads to the formation of insoluble fibrin polymers.

## Serum

**Serum** is defined as the fluid portion of blood remaining after clotting factors and cellular elements have been removed. When blood is drawn, it clots within minutes when left undisturbed. This complex process involves a number of steps (outlined in figure 3.2). Both disintegration of platelets and tissue trauma initiate steps that lead to the formation of the enzyme, prothrombinase. When platelets are destroyed, a substance is released that reacts with divalent calcium ions and other plasma proteins to form prothrombinase. Traumatized tissue releases thromboplastin (a lipoprotein) that also reacts with calcium and plasma proteins to form prothrombinase. Prothrombin, a protein released from the liver, is hydrolyzed by prothrombinase in the presence of calcium to form another proteolytic enzyme called thrombin. At this point, fibrinogen is degraded by thrombin to produce fibrin. Fibrin becomes arranged into long threads arranged into a meshwork.

Obviously, blood clotting results from an intricate and complex series of reactions. This is also true of all aspects of the **immune response** but, unlike the process of clotting of blood, the details of the immune response remain somewhat unclear. Immunologists in the future face the challenge of presenting a clear picture of the interrelationships of immune cells and molecules.

The polymeric fibrin network is referred to as a **clot** and, when formed, encloses all the blood cells within itself. When blood is refrigerated, the clot shrinks more, forcing out a clear, straw-colored serum. Serum can be collected and preserved by refrigeration.

The addition of **anticoagulants,** such as sodium citrate, heparin or potassium oxalate, can inhibit the clotting process. These interfere with clotting by removing calcium ions, making them unavailable for the formation of thrombin. After centrifugation of freshly drawn blood that has been treated with an anticoagulant, a clear liquid containing fibrinogen can be withdrawn, and this is termed **plasma.**

Plasma contains a significant amount of protein, perhaps as much as 10%. Plasma proteins, categorized as albumins, globulins and fibrinogen, can be separated by electrophoresis or by solubility characteristics.

Electrophoresis (discussed in exercise 9) separates serum proteins into at least four fractions: (1) albumin, (2) alpha globulin, (3) beta globulin, and (4) gamma globulin. These fractions can be further characterized. Globulins are necessary for osmotic regulation of body fluids and tissues. In addition, they play an important role in cell nutrition. **Gamma globulin** fractions contain antibodies—proteins that have the unique ability to react specifically with the antigen that caused the formation of the antibody. Many tests have been devised to measure the presence and concentration of antibodies in serum.

## Blood Cells

Blood contains several cellular elements with many different functions. All have a limited life span and are continually renewed from **hematopoietic stem cells** that give rise to all of the differentiated blood cells. These stem cells are therefore pluripotent, and the process of differentiation is termed **hematopoiesis.** It occurs in the bone marrow and

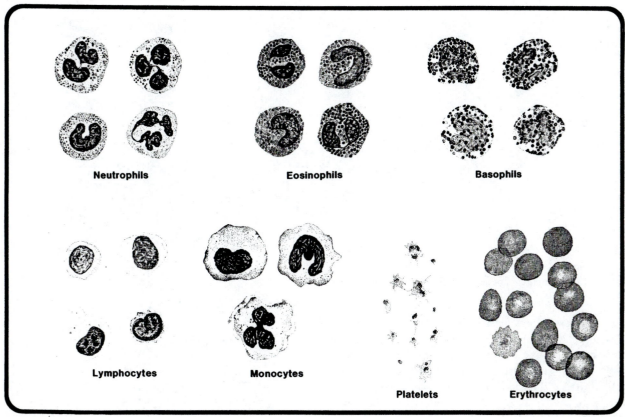

**FIGURE 3.3**
The cellular elements of the blood.

K. P. Talaro

From Harold J. Benson, et al., *Anatomy and Physiology Laboratory Textbook*, Complete Version, 4th ed. Copyright © 1988 Wm. C. Brown Publishers, Dubuque, Iowa. All Rights Reserved. Reprinted by permission.

**Table 3.1**  White Blood Cells

| Type | Function | Appearance (After Wright's Staining) |
|---|---|---|
| Neutrophil | Phagocytic | Lobed (2–5 lobes) nucleus with lobes connected by thin filaments. Color may be dark blue or purple. Cytoplasm is lilac with fine, deep lilac-colored granules. |
| Eosinophil | Detoxifying; secretes enzymes | Nucleus usually has 2 lobes that stain blue-red or blue. Cytoplasm is pale lilac with large, deep pink granules of equal size. |
| Basophil | Releases heparin | Slightly polymorph nucleus that stains pale blue. The cytoplasm is pink, and granules are coarse and equal sized. There are only a few granules, and they stain deep bluish-purple. |
| Monocyte | Phagocytic | Nucleus is "bean-shaped." Stains pale blue. Cytoplasm is gray-blue with non-specific granules that are not easily seen. |
| Lymphocyte | Provides immune response | Round nucleus that is not easily distinguished from the cytoplasm and stains dark blue. Cytoplasm is small but clear blue. Granules are not visible. |

involves a complicated series of reactions that results in a balanced number of each cell type.

Blood cells can easily be seen and differentiated as red or white. Red cells are **erythrocytes,** and white cells are **leukocytes.** The major function of erythrocytes is to transport oxygen throughout the body using hemoglobin. Leukocytes are responsible for resistance to infection. They either engulf foreign materials, produce substances detrimental to invading agents of disease, or react directly with other cells. Another cell fragment found in blood is the platelet, an important component in the clotting of blood as described above.

Red blood cells and platelets are not divided into morphological groups. However, white blood cells form **five**

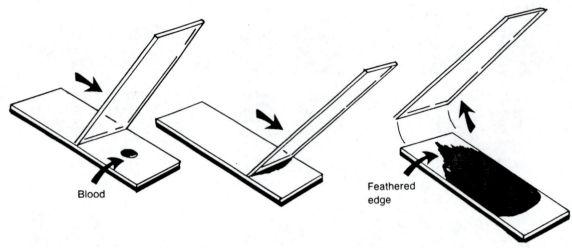

Blood

Feathered
edge

**FIGURE 3.4**
The procedure for preparing a thin blood smear for staining.

**different classes.** Each class is distinguished from all others by morphological characteristics as seen using a light microscope. The five classes and percentages of each include: (1) neutrophil (also called polymorphonuclear leukocyte), 50–70%; (2) eosinophil, 1–5%; (3) basophil, 0.5–1%; (4) lymphocyte, 20–30%; and (5) monocyte, 2–6%. Certain leukocytes contain granules in their cytoplasm. These, collectively called **granulocytes,** include neutrophils, eosinophils and basophils.

Lymphocytes are especially important to the immunologist because of the role they play in the immune response. Lymphocytes, the true immune cells, functionally respond to foreign substances. Lymphocytes can easily be isolated, fractionated, and characterized.

Neutrophils destroy invading bacteria. Eosinophils may destroy parasites and become involved in allergic and inflammatory reactions; basophils release heparin, histamine and pharmacological mediators of immune reactions. Lymphocytes are involved in both humoral and cell-mediated immune reactions. Monocytes may differentiate into macrophages in tissue, and these cells help process antigen and present it to lymphocytes. Important morphological characteristics of these major classes of cells appear in figure 3.3 and are described in table 3.1 by appearance after Wright's staining.

## MATERIALS

(Per pair)

1 hemacytometer (improved Neubauer chamber)
1 Unopette® white cell test (including diluting fluid and reservoir)
Alcohol swabs

Lancets
Microscope slides
Wright's stain
Wright's buffer
Hand counter
Microscope

## PROCEDURE

Blood cell counts (both red and white) help to determine the physiological well-being of the individual. Counting can be done manually or with electronic particle counters. The electronic particle counters are also used to count cells in some body fluids such as cerebrospinal, synovial and pericardial fluids. A popular instrument used in the hematology laboratory is the Coulter® STKS, a quantitative, automated hematology analyzer and leukocyte differential counter. It performs a complete blood count and a differential white blood cell count. The results can identify abnormal cells or counts in an individual. Additional tests such as a manual white blood cell count could be indicated. Normal human blood contains between $4.2 \times 10^6$ and $5.4 \times 10^6$ erythrocytes/mm$^3$ and $5 \times 10^3$ to $8 \times 10^3$ leukocytes/mm$^3$.

A **differential** white blood cell count is used to determine the percentages of different types of white blood cells present. It can determine the presence of disease since the proportion of cell types may indicate a particular disease. For example, neutrophils may increase during bacterial disease, and eosinophils may increase during certain allergic disorders.

## Note

The use (study) of human blood in clinical situations or in the experimental laboratory poses problems that must be addressed. Blood (and other body fluids) should be considered **potential health hazards** due to the possibility of contamination with the hepatitis B surface antigen (HBsAg), the human immunodeficiency virus (HIV–1) or a number of bacterial pathogens. The **Centers for Disease Control and Prevention** stresses the need to enforce recommendations for minimizing the risk of exposure to blood and body fluids. Individuals working with blood should always wear latex gloves and properly dispose of blood. Never mouth pipette blood or blood products. Also see safety rules in exercise 17. To minimize exposure in this exercise, the Unopette® method will be used to determine a total white blood cell count. This system, designed to provide standardized collection, pipetting and dilutions of small blood samples with a minimum of handling, also eliminates the need for mouth pipetting.

## Total White Blood Cell Count

1. Cleanse your left middle finger thoroughly with 70% ethanol.
2. Prick the clean area with a sterile lancet and squeeze your finger to produce a drop of blood. Discard the first drop.
3. Draw the blood up to the appropriate mark on the Unopette® pipette used with the white cell test. The diluting fluid is included with the test. See the appendix for the composition of white blood cell diluting fluid. Follow directions for mixing the diluting fluid and blood.
4. Shake the reservoir horizontally for 1 to 2 min.
5. Discard the first 3 or 4 drops and then fill the chamber of a hemacytometer via capillary attraction. If the chamber is overfilled, clean and refill it.
6. Allow the cells to settle for approximately 1 min.
7. Using the 10× objective of the microscope, count the number of white blood cells in the four large corner squares of the ruled area of the hemacytometer (sections A, B, C and D in figure 1.3).
8. Multiply the total number obtained by 50 (the conversion factor) to determine the total number of white blood cells/mm$^3$ of blood. See the appendix for an explanation of the conversion factor.

## Differential White Blood Cell Count

1. Secure two clean microscope slides.
2. Using the procedure described for preparing and puncturing the finger, place a drop of blood at one end of a microscope slide.
3. With another slide prepare a thin, even blood smear in the following manner:
   a. Place the other slide (spreader slide) at a 30 degree angle and touch the slide that has the drop of blood.
   b. Move the spreader slide along until the edge touches the drop of blood. Notice that capillarity spreads the blood along the edge.
   c. Immediately pull the spreader slide away from the drop of blood and notice that the blood makes a thin smear that dries immediately. A "feathered edge" on the smear indicates that the technique was done properly (see figure 3.4).
4. Stain the smear with Wright's stain using the following method:
   a. Add 15 drops of Wright's stain to the blood smear. Allow the stain to remain in contact with the smear for 5 min. Gently blow across the stain 3 or 4 times during the staining period. See the appendix for the formulation of Wright's stain.
   b. Add 15 drops of distilled water or Wright's buffer directly to the staining solution on the smear. If the buffer is used, let it remain until a green metallic sheen appears on the surface (approximately 2 min).
   c. Wash away the stain and the buffer, if used, with distilled water. Continue to wash until the smear appears pink.
   d. Air dry.
   e. Observe with the oil immersion objective. The erythrocytes will appear pink, and each white blood cell will have a purple nucleus.
   f. Count and classify 100 white blood cells using figure 3.3 and table 3.1 as guides.

## DISCUSSION

Although more than 60% of the requests for total white blood cell counts and differential white blood cell counts are done with automated instruments like the one described above, the methods presented here are accurate when performed properly. However, the possibility for experimental error certainly exists. The major problems encountered involve accurate diluting (including pipetting) and counting.

## SELECTED REFERENCES

Bryant, N. J. 1982. *An introduction to hematology.* 2d ed. Philadelphia, PA: W. B. Saunders Co.

Quesenberry, P., and L. Levitt. 1979. Hematopoietic stem cells. *N. Eng. J. Med.* 301(14):755.

Sacho, Leo. 1987. The molecular control of blood cell development. *Science.* 238:1374.

Walker, R. H., ed. 1990. *Technical Manual.* Arlington, VA: American Association of Blood Banks.

Zucker-Franklin, D., M. F. Greaves, C. E. Grossi and A. M. Marmont. 1988. *Atlas of blood cells: Function and pathology.* 2d ed. Philadelphia, PA: Lea and Febiger.

# Natural Resistance to Infection

## INTRODUCTION

**Natural resistance** is a term used to explain the resistance and resistance factors that are inherently available to protect an individual from infectious disease. People are born with most of these factors and, therefore, do not acquire them because of exposure to an infectious agent. Other terms used to describe natural resistance are **innate resistance** and **innate immunity.** Natural resistance factors are nonspecific—equally effective against many different invading microorganisms and viruses. The student should compare natural resistance or innate resistance to acquired immunity.

The effectiveness of natural resistance to infection depends upon a number of factors, including the physiological well-being of the individual. A person's state of health varies from time to time as a result of exposure to temperature extremes, poor nutrition, drug use, mental status, and other things. Any factor that disrupts the ability of natural resistance factors to function properly predisposes the individual to infectious disease. The human body possesses a number of these remarkable nonspecific resistance mechanisms (figure 4.1).

The first barrier encountered by an invading microorganism is the **skin.** Few bacteria can survive for very long on the surface of the skin due to the presence of lactic acid and fatty acids in sebaceous secretions. *Staphylococcus aureus* may be one exception, however, because it may infect hair follicles and glands. The intact skin is probably impermeable to microorganisms, and only when the skin is broken is the barrier to infection broken.

The **presence of mucus,** another defense mechanism, coats the inner membrane surfaces of the body and serves as a protective barrier for cells comprising membranes.

Viruses as well as microorganisms cannot penetrate the mucus film, or are inactivated by it. They are subsequently removed from the body as they are swept away in mucus by ciliary activity of cells.

Other **body fluids contain substances** that are detrimental to microbial invasion. The list of fluids includes tears, urine, gastric juice, and saliva. Tears, as well as other body fluids, contain lysozyme which degrades the peptidoglycan molecule of some bacterial cell walls.

Lysozyme is only one of a number of humoral, nonspecific, antimicrobial substances found in body fluids. Another important group of substances, collectively called **complement,** appears in serum and participates in: (1) an antigen-antibody mediated series of reactions called the **classical pathway,** and (2) an **alternate pathway** that does not involve antibody or other components of the immune system. The classical complement pathway is comprised of components numbered C1 through C9. Most of these are beta-globulins with molecular weights around 200,000. C1 fixation occurs when certain classes of immunoglobulin (such as IgG and IgM) react with antigen. Other complement components then react with this complex in a cascading manner to produce immunological activities. These include activation of immune cells (e.g., macrophage), cytolysis of target cells, and neutralization of the antiphagocytic property of the bacterial capsule (opsonization).

The alternate pathway is not antigen-specific and therefore cannot be considered an immune phenomenon. It is a natural response to invading cells. The alternate pathway is initiated with the deposition of the C3b complement fragment on an invading cell. The pathway is then activated and terminates with the same results as the classical pathway.

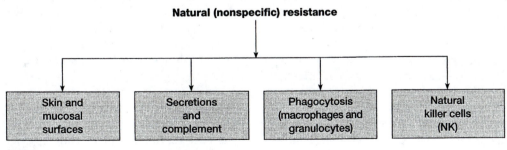

**FIGURE 4.1**
Some examples of natural resistance factors.

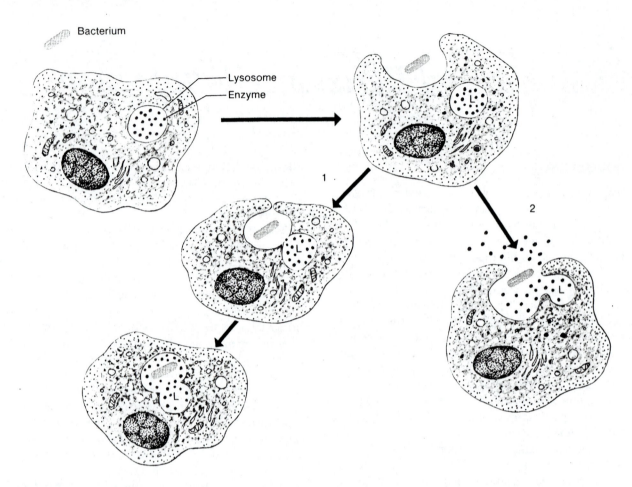

**FIGURE 4.2**
Phagocytosis by a leukocyte. A phagocytic cell extends its pseudopods around the object to be engulfed (such as the bacterium shown). Dots represent lysosomal enzymes (L = lysosome). If the pseudopods fuse to form a complete vacuole (1), lysosomal enzymes are released into the vacuole. If the lysosome fuses with the vacuole before the pseudopods fuse (2), lysosomal enzymes are released into the surrounding tissue.

From Stuart Ira Fox, *Human Physiology*, 2d ed. Copyright © 1987 Wm. C. Brown Publishers, Dubuque, Iowa. All Rights Reserved. Reprinted by permission.

Humoral factors responsible for death of Gram-negative bacteria include properdin (found in serum) and phagocytin (produced by phagocytic cells). Many serum proteins such as C-reactive protein (CRP), alpha-1-antitrypsin, alpha-2-macroglobulin, fibrinogen, and others possess antibacterial properties. These proteins increase in concentration during the acute phase of many infections. Humoral substances specifically responsible for killing of Gram-positive bacteria include betalysin, leukin (produced by leukocytes), and basic proteins like protamine.

One substance that possesses antiviral activity is **interferon.** It inhibits intracellular viral replication. Interferon is synthesized by cells in response to a virus, and other cells are protected from infection by the same virus or other unrelated viruses by the action of interferon.

Another natural resistance mechanism, **phagocytosis,** involves a process whereby macrophages and neutrophils engulf foreign materials, cellular debris, and microorganisms (figure 4.2). Macrophages are strategically located in tissue throughout the body, including connective tissue,

basement membrane of small blood vessels, lung, liver, spleen and lymph nodes. After the ingestion process is complete, the phagocytized material is contained within a vacuole. A lysosome, containing hydrolytic and proteolytic enzymes, fuses with the vacuole. An entire battery of digestive enzymes then destroys the ingested material.

A burst of oxidative reactions accompanies the digestive process. A measurable increase in hexose monophosphate shunt activity produces NADPH with a concomitant utilization of oxygen. Oxygen is converted to a variety of microbicidal substances including superoxide anion, hydrogen peroxide, singlet oxygen and hydroxyl radicals.

Not all ingested microorganisms and viruses are destroyed by the phagocytic cell, and some bacteria can even reproduce within the macrophage. **Intracellular pathogens** can survive within a phagocytic cell or other host cell where they are hidden from the phagocytic cell.

This exercise explores natural resistance to bacterial infection. The first part of the exercise determines the effectiveness of the **endoreticular system** in eliminating microorganisms from the blood. The endoreticular system is a network of large mononuclear cells associated with reticular fibers found in many organs of the body. One important function of this system is phagocytosis. A predetermined number of *Escherichia coli,* a Gram-negative bacterium which may cause bacteremia, will be injected intravenously into a rabbit. At specific time intervals, blood samples will be taken and bacterial colony-forming units (CFU) determined. A reduction in CFU in blood with time will indicate elimination of bacteria by cells specifically designed for this purpose.

The other part of this exercise allows observation of in vitro phagocytosis. Phagocytic cells will be maintained in culture. A specific number of *Bacillus cereus* cells (or other bacteria chosen by the instructor) will be added to cultured phagocytic cells and incubated. After a predetermined time interval, a Wright's stain and microscopic examination will show bacteria within phagocytes.

## MATERIALS

A. Removal of Bacteria by the Endoreticular System
   (Per class)

   1 18- to 24-hr culture of *Escherichia coli* in BHIB

   11 9.0-ml sterile saline blanks

   12 BHIA deeps

   12 sterile Petri dishes

   1 hemacytometer

   1 rabbit

   1 tuberculin needle and syringe

   3 6-ml syringes with 18-gauge needles (for cardiac puncture)

   Razor or single-edge razor blade and soap

   1-ml pipettes

   Sterile surgical instruments

   Heparin

   70% ethanol

   Hand counter

   50° C water bath

   Ketamine hydrochloride (for rabbit anesthesia)

B. In Vitro Phagocytosis
   (Per 4 students)

   1 18-hr culture *Bacillus cereus* in BHIB

   3 9.0-ml saline blanks

   1 bottle Eagle's Minimal Essential Medium (EMEM, perhaps referred to as Basal Medium Eagle, prewarmed to 37° C)

   2 sterile 13 × 100-mm test tubes

   $CO_2$ for mouse euthanasia

1 mouse (6–8 wk old)

1 hemacytometer

1 12-ml syringe with 21-gauge needle

1 20-ml syringe with 18-gauge needle

1 microscope slide

1 sterile plastic Petri dish

Centrifuge with swinging bucket rotor

Wright's stain and buffer

Hand counter

Pipettes and tubes for dilution series

## PROCEDURE

## Removal of Bacteria by the Endoreticular System

1. This experiment will be performed as a class exercise. Several students will take part by performing various tasks.
2. Brain heart infusion agar (BHIA) deeps have been melted and tempered to 50° C. Sterile Petri dishes are available.
3. Dilute a suspension of *E. coli* to $10^8$ cells/ml (count using a hemacytometer as described in exercise 1). Use saline as the diluent throughout.
4. Anesthetize the rabbit with ketamine using the procedure outlined in exercise 1 or as directed by the instructor.
5. Inject 1 ml of the diluted bacteria into the marginal ear vein of a rabbit using techniques described in exercise 1.
6. With a syringe and needle containing heparin or other anticoagulant, **immediately** withdraw 2 to 3 ml of blood from the heart or the marginal ear vein (the instructor may perform this step). Use accepted procedures described in exercise 1. For this exercise the student only needs to draw heparin into the needle and then expel it to provide enough heparin to prevent clotting of 2 to 3 ml of blood.
7. Make $10^{-2}$ through $10^{-6}$ dilutions of the blood sample and plate each using BHIA. To do this prepare the proper dilutions of blood and pipette 1 ml of the correct dilution of blood into a sterile Petri dish, pour the BHIA into the dish and swirl gently. Allow to solidify and incubate. Properly label all plates.
8. At the end of 15 min once again draw 3 ml of blood from the heart and plate the $10^{-1}$ through $10^{-4}$ dilutions.

9. At the end of 30 min draw an additional 3 ml of blood and plate a $10^{-1}$ dilution and also plate 1 ml of undiluted blood.
10. Incubate all plates for 24 to 48 hr at 37° C and count colony-forming units (CFU).
11. Prepare a graph that indicates clearance of bacteria from the blood after specific periods of time.

## In Vitro Phagocytosis

1. This experiment should be carried out by groups of four students. Each individual should take an active part in the procedure. Prepare all materials used in this experiment and have them ready to use before proceeding.
2. Prepare a saline suspension of an 18-hr culture of *B. cereus* with $10^6$ cells/ml (use a hemacytometer as previously described).
3. Kill a mouse with carbon dioxide ($CO_2$) asphyxiation. To do this, place the animal in a closed container with 70 to 100% $CO_2$. Tank $CO_2$ may be used, or it may be generated with dry ice. Alternatively, the animal can be killed with a pentobarbital overdose. Inject 60 mg/kg intraperitoneally. Verify death by observing fixed and dilated pupils before continuing.
4. Inject 8 ml of prewarmed (37° C) Eagles Minimal Essential Medium (EMEM) intraperitoneally. Follow the procedure for intraperitoneal injection given in exericse 1 and prepare EMEM according to the formulation listed in the appendix or according to the manufacturer's instructions.
5. Massage the abdominal area for 1 min to suspend peritoneal cells.
6. Carefully withdraw the EMEM and **suspended cells** from the peritoneal cavity with an 18-gauge needle on a 20-ml syringe. The suspended cells will be referred to as **peritoneal exudate cells** (PEC) and are primarily macrophages and lymphocytes. For best results the suspension should be free of erythrocytes.
7. Dispense the PEC suspension into a clean and sterile 13 × 100-mm tube and centrifuge at 1,000 × g for 5 min.
8. Decant the supernatant and add 8 ml of prewarmed EMEM. Resuspend the pelleted PEC by gently vortexing.
9. Place a thoroughly **cleaned** (remove all residual detergent, etc.) glass microscope slide into a sterile, plastic Petri dish and pour the PEC suspension into the dish to cover the slide. Incubate for 30 min at 37° C.
10. After incubation, decant the EMEM and gently wash the slide with warm EMEM. The macrophages will adhere to the glass microscope slide, and other cells will be washed away. Put the slide in a new dish and add an additional 8 ml of EMEM. Do not allow the slide to dry during this procedure.
11. Carefully pipette 1 ml of the suspension of *B. cereus* into the dish and incubate for an additional 30 min.
12. Remove the slide, wash once with EMEM, and allow to air dry.
13. Stain with Wright's stain as described in exercise 3.
14. Observe the stained phagocytes microscopically for the presence of intracellular, rod-shaped bacteria.
15. Record the observations.

## DISCUSSION

The first part of this exercise works best when duplicate or triplicate plates are prepared. Some individuals prefer spread plates to pour plates for bacterial enumeration. Spread plates would work well in this procedure and may actually save time by eliminating dispensing of agar into tubes.

The experiment designed to show phagocytosis does not distinguish between adherence of the bacteria to the phagocytic cell and actual phagocytosis. Adherence (or binding) precedes phagocytosis; however, phagocytosis does not necessarily follow binding. More sophisticated techniques have been devised to determine whether phagocytosis is occurring.

Select a method for euthanasia of the mouse that does not affect the cells to be studied. Either method described here works well for this experiment. Carbon dioxide can easily be generated by placing dry ice in warm water in a sealed container. The mouse is placed in the container on a platform (bent wire mesh) above the dry ice to prevent contact. Security is important if pentobarbital (sodium pentobarbital) is used because it is a controlled substance. Finally, the instructor may decide to use cervical dislocation.

## SELECTED REFERENCES

Albright, J. F., and J. W. Albright. 1984. Natural resistance to animal parasites. *Contemp. Topics Immunobiol.* 12:1.

Came, P. E., and W. A. Carter, eds. 1984. *Interferons and their applications.* Berlin: Springer-Verlag.

Elsbach, P. 1980. Degradation of microorganisms by phagocytic cells. *Rev. Inf. Dis.* 2:106.

Fox, J. G., B. J. Cohen, and F. M. Lowe, eds. 1984. *Laboratory Animal Medicine.* Orlando, FL: Academic Press.

Freidman, R. M., and S. N. Vogel. 1983. Interferons with special emphasis on the immune system. *Adv. Immunol.* 34:97.

Geisow, M. 1980. Pathways of endocytosis. *Nature.* 288:434.

Hirst, R. L. 1982. The complement system: Its importance to host response to viral infection. *Microbiol. Rev.* 46:71.

Oppenheim, J., and D. Jacobs, eds. 1986. *Leukocytes and host defense.* New York, NY: Allan R. Liss, Inc.

*Assay
Procedures*

Procedures that help to detect and quantitate products of the immune system are basic to most immunology laboratories. Even the most sophisticated and complex laboratory relies on fundamental **assay techniques.** The exercises presented in section II teach these techniques and reinforce theoretical concepts of assay procedures presented in textbooks.

The first exercise guides the student through a procedure designed to determine the **titer of an antiserum.** The procedure is written so, that by carefully following instructions, the student will detect a soluble antibody indicated by a visible precipitation. The first part makes use of the ring interfacial test for an estimation of titer, and the second part uses information from the ring interfacial test to determine the actual ratio of antigen to antibody required to form **equivalence.** Although at first glance the procedure appears easy to follow, many students have difficulty putting the directions into practice. For that reason **diagrams** (or flow sheets) of the experimental design are provided.

After gaining experience with precipitation reactions, the student will construct a **precipitation curve.** A purified protein is used to produce a protein **standard curve** using the spectrophotometric Bradford or Lowry method. The sediments (precipitated antigen and antibody) from the previous exercise are analyzed for protein content as determined from the standard curve. The results should be interpreted in view of the amount of antigen and antibody that was available in each reaction tube in the previous exercise. A better understanding of antigen-antibody reactions will result.

The next exercise studies **particulate antigens** and reactions with antibody to produce **agglutination.** Human blood grouping is an excellent procedure to use as an example of agglutination phenomena. After blood grouping, a study of bacterial agglutination antibodies reinforces the agglutination concept. The **slide** and **tube tests** detect and quantitate antibodies to *Salmonella* species.

A considerable number of in vitro **agglutination tests** are clinically useful in the diagnosis of various human diseases. Several of these, presented in this section, demonstrate to students the application of an **immunologic assay.** A discussion of the mechanisms involved in each test accompanies the exercise. All of the tests suggested can be purchased from manufacturers as kits for the in vitro diagnosis of disease.

**Electrophoresis** is the subject of exercise 9, and the applications referred to and studied follow the theme of the previous exercise, that is, the diagnosis of human disease. Students will electrophorese human serum and see the method as a diagnostic tool. Figures from the literature that contain relevant information are provided, and an extension of this method is presented in another section.

The final exercise in section II is a method for assaying antigen-antibody reactions in gel. It presents both **single** and **double diffusion techniques.** The Ouchterlony double diffusion method introduces the student to gel diffusion. The second part of the exercise provides an application of the technique. This application, the Mancini single diffusion technique, is used clinically as a quantitative measure of serum antibody. All materials used are available commercially.

*The approximate instructor preparation time and student laboratory time necessary for successful completion of exercises 5 through 10 are presented in figure II.*

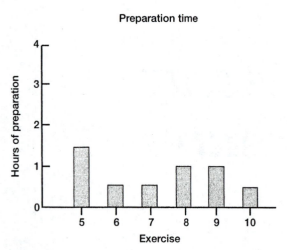

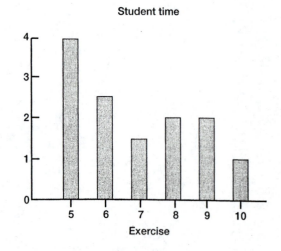

**FIGURE II**
Time allocation for Section II exercises.

# EXERCISE

# 5

# *Precipitation*

## INTRODUCTION

Soluble antigens that react in vitro with homologous antibodies produce a visible reaction called **precipitation.** The antigens involved in these reactions may be derived from several sources such as microorganisms (bacteria and fungi), viruses, plants and animals. Procedures to measure the amount of precipitating antigen (or antibody) in solution can be either qualitative or quantitative. This exercise provides a procedure for precipitating bovine serum albumin (BSA) with anti-BSA.

The lattice hypothesis states that soluble antigens react in vitro with precipitating antibodies to form a **lattice** or framework composed of alternating antigen and antibody molecules. The theory assumes that both reactants are at least divalent (antigens are usually multivalent) and that the antibodies act as bridges to link antigens together. Such a structure results in a large insoluble aggregate of antigens and antibodies that eventually becomes sufficiently large to become visible. Upon standing, the aggregate can settle to the bottom of a tube. This phenomenon is called **precipitation.**

This interaction of reactants requires optimal conditions to occur. The **proper concentration** of both antigen and antibody is necessary and is considered the most critical condition that must be met to produce insoluble aggregates. **Optimal proportions** (equivalent proportions) of each result in usage of all available antigen and antibody in formation of the lattice. To produce optimal proportions of each, dilution is usually necessary. Depending upon the result desired, either the antigen or antibody may be diluted, but dilution of antigen is the most common procedure.

When equivalent proportions of antigen and antibody are mixed and incubated, addition of more antigen or antibody to the supernatant will produce no additional precipitation. The reason is that all reactants participated in the initial reaction. This is the ideal situation, and many tests have been designed to obtain this result. When **excess antibody** is added to a reaction mixture, all of the epitopes on the antigen are covered by antibody resulting in inhibition of lattice formation. **Excess antigen** has a similar effect since there will not be sufficient antibody to crosslink with antigen to form the lattice, and once again, precipitation is inhibited.

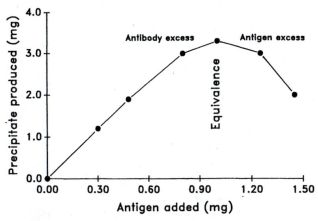

**FIGURE 5.1**
A precipitation curve. Diluted antigen was added to constant amounts of antibody, and the quantity of precipitate was measured.

The problem is, therefore, to determine the optimal concentration of both antigen and antibody. This is accomplished by serial dilution of antigen and addition of these dilutions to **constant amounts** of antibody. The amount of precipitation that results can be measured visually or chemically, and the dilution of antigen that gives the greatest amount of precipitation is considered to be **equivalence.**

Figure 5.1 represents a typical protein **precipitation curve.** To produce the curve, specific amounts (mg) of antigen were added to a series of tubes, each containing a constant amount of antibody. After an incubation period sufficient to allow all components to react, the precipitate was collected and assayed. The amounts of precipitate were plotted against the amounts of antigen added, and this produced the precipitation curve.

To determine which tube contains excess antigen or antibody, the **supernatant fractions** could be further studied. To portions of each supernatant, more antigen or antibody could be added and the tubes observed for additional precipitation. The tube that shows no additional precipitation when either antigen or antibody is added is by definition the **equivalence point** of the precipitation curve.

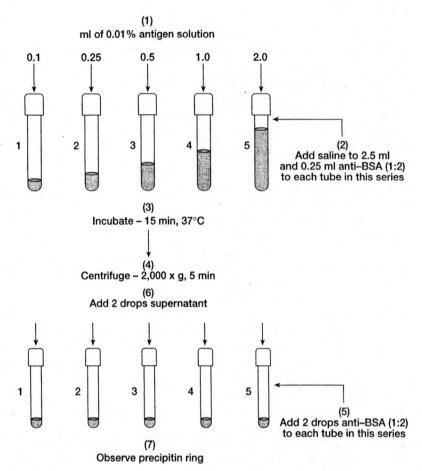

**(1)**
ml of 0.01% antigen solution

0.1    0.25    0.5    1.0    2.0

**(2)**
Add saline to 2.5 ml
and 0.25 ml anti–BSA (1:2)
to each tube in this series

**(3)**
Incubate – 15 min, 37°C

**(4)**
Centrifuge – 2,000 x g, 5 min

**(6)**
Add 2 drops supernatant

**(5)**
Add 2 drops anti–BSA (1:2)
to each tube in this series

**(7)**
Observe precipitin ring

**FIGURE 5.2**
Titration of antiserum. A flow diagram for the procedure to determine the amount of
antigen needed for maximum in vitro precipitation of antibody.

## MATERIALS

(Per pair)

Anti-BSA (diluted 1:2)

0.01% BSA

Saline

Capillary pipettes

9 13 × 100-mm tubes

13 6 × 50-mm tubes

Pipettes (1- and 5-ml)

37° C water bath

Centrifuge

## PROCEDURE

1. The first procedure teaches the student how to
   determine the antibody titer of the sample.
   Before starting, a preliminary test, the titration
   of antiserum, must be run to determine the
   **approximate dilutions** of antibody to be used.

## Titration of Antiserum (figure 5.2)

a. Carefully pipette 0.25 ml of anti-BSA
   (diluted 1:2) into each of 5, 13 × 100-mm
   tubes placed in a rack. Number the tubes.

b. Pipette 0.1 ml of 0.01% BSA into tube 1, 0.25
   into 2, 0.5 into 3, 1.0 into 4, and 2.0 ml into 5.
   What are the resulting dilutions of BSA?
   Save the remaining antigen for use later.

c. Add sufficient saline to each tube to give a
   total of 2.5 ml.

d. Mix **thoroughly** and incubate for 15 min in a
   water bath at 37° C.

e. Centrifuge for 5 min at 2,000 × g.

f. Pipette 2 drops of anti-BSA (1:2 dilution) into
   each of 5, clean 6 × 50 mm tubes with a capillary pipette. Number the tubes. **Carefully overlay** each tube of anti-BSA with 2 drops of
   supernatant that was produced from each dilution
   above. For example, put 2 drops from tube 1 in
   the first series of tubes into tube 1 of the second
   series of tubes, 2 drops from tube 2 in the first
   series to tube 2 of the second series, etc.

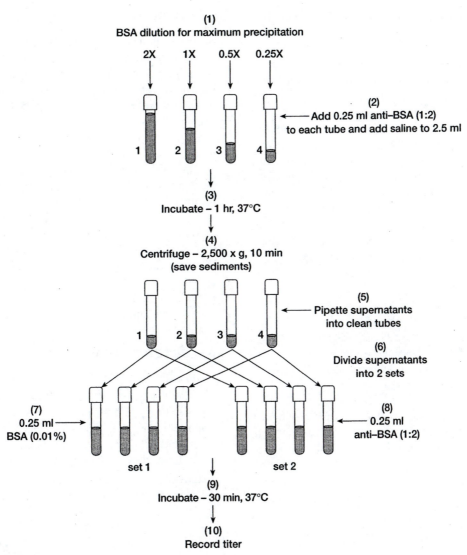

**(1)**
BSA dilution for maximum precipitation

2X    1X    0.5X    0.25X

1    2    3    4

**(2)**
Add 0.25 ml anti–BSA (1:2)
to each tube and add saline to 2.5 ml

**(3)**
Incubate – 1 hr, 37°C

**(4)**
Centrifuge – 2,500 x g, 10 min
(save sediments)

1    2    3    4

**(5)**
Pipette supernatants
into clean tubes

**(6)**
Divide supernatants
into 2 sets

**(7)**
0.25 ml
BSA (0.01%)

**(8)**
0.25 ml
anti–BSA (1:2)

set 1        set 2

**(9)**
Incubate – 30 min, 37°C

**(10)**
Record titer

**FIGURE 5.3**
A flow diagram for the procedure to show the presence of excess antigen or antibody. The
equivalence point can be determined from this exercise.

g. Look for formation of a ring of precipitate at
the interface of antigen and antibody that
occurs within 15 min.

h. **Results:**
 1) Choose the tube that has a ring of
 precipitate at the interface. This
 represents an **antigen excess.** Why?
 2) If precipitate occurs in all tubes, the test
 must be repeated using smaller amounts
 of antigen.
 3) If no precipitate occurs, antigen excess
 was not reached.
 4) This procedure has established the
 amount of antigen needed for maximum
 precipitation and is necessary to proceed
 to Step 2.

## Determination of Equivalence (figure 5.3)

 2. Set up a series of 4 tubes (13 × 100 mm).
 3. To the first add twice the amount of antigen
 determined above to give maximum
 precipitation. For example, if supernatant from
 the tube above with 1.0 ml of antigen gave an
 antigen-excess reaction, then the tube with
 0.5 ml of antigen should give maximum
 precipitation. Therefore, one would add 1 ml
 (twice the amount) to tube 1. To the second tube
 add the exact amount needed; to the third, one-
 half this amount; to the fourth, one-quarter this
 amount.
 4. Add 0.25 ml of the 1:2 dilution of anti-BSA
 antiserum to each tube.

5.  Add enough saline to make a total of 2.5 ml. Mix.
6.  Incubate in a water bath at 37° C for 1 hr. For **maximum results,** the mixture can be further incubated in the cold with frequent shaking for 48 hr.
7.  Centrifuge all tubes for 10 min at 2,500 × g. Again, for maximum results, all centrifugations should be done in the cold.
8.  Carefully remove the supernatant from each tube with a capillary pipette and save in a clean tube. Be careful not to lose any of the sediment. Cap or seal the tubes with plastic wrap and save the sediments in the cold room for use in exercise 6.
9.  From each of the 4 supernatants pipette approximately 0.25 ml with a capillary pipette into each of 2, 6 × 50-mm tubes. This will produce 2 sets of 4 tubes.
10. To each tube of one set add approximately 0.25 ml of BSA (0.01%).
11. To each tube of the other set add approximately 0.25 ml of anti-BSA (1:2 dilution).
12. Incubate all tubes in a water bath at 37° C for 30 min. and look for precipitation.
13. Record the tube that has a slight excess of antigen. The results should show precipitate in the last tube(s) of one set when antigen is added, and in the first tube(s) of the second set when antibody is added. Explain.

## DISCUSSION

Experiments such as the one described here require the student to plan ahead and utilize the time allotted wisely. Flow sheets and diagrams are very useful and help the student follow directions so that at the completion of the exercise, meaningful results are obtained. Flow diagrams such as the ones presented in this exercise should be prepared by the student prior to the laboratory period for all subsequent procedures.

This procedure also requires good laboratory technique. By this time in the semester, the student will have mastered techniques that will be used again in the following exercises.

As defined, the equilibrium point is the point where neither antigen nor antibody causes any additional precipitate. However, note that this point does not necessarily correspond to the **exact point** of maximum precipitation. It may occur to the left of equilibrium on the precipitation curve when studied in critical and sensitive experiments. Why?

## SELECTED REFERENCES

Harlow, E., and D. Lane. 1988. *Antibodies: A laboratory manual.* Cold Spring Harbor, NY: Cold Spring Harbor Laboratory.

Landsteiner, K. 1945. *The specificity of serologic reactions.* Harvard University Press. Cambridge. Revised ed. 1962. New York, NY: Dover Press Inc.

Letkovits, I., and B. Pernis, eds. 1985. *Immunological methods.* Vol. 1–3. Orlando, FL: Academic Press.

# *Precipitation Curve*

## INTRODUCTION

This exercise will produce data to construct a **precipitation curve** (or calibration curve). The student will use the precipitate and principles of precipitation formation that were developed in exercise 5. The curve will result from assaying the protein content of the precipitate by measuring absorbance after color development using either the Bradford or Lowry method.

The Bradford method, a reliable method for protein determinations, can be rapidly completed. It relies upon binding the dye, Coomassie Brilliant Blue, to protein. When proteins are dissolved in an acid-alcoholic medium, they will react with the dye. A blue color results which can be read in a spectrophotometer at $A_{595}$. Protein concentrations in the range of 10 to 100 µg can easily be detected.

The Lowry method (Folin-Ciocalteu) is also a colorimetric quantitation of soluble proteins. Also sensitive, it will detect proteins at a level as low as 5 µg. Alkaline cupric tartrate reagent complexes with peptide bonds to produce a purple-blue color when the phenol reagent is added. The resulting color depends specifically upon the tryptophan and tyrosine content of the protein.

For any assay of this type, data derived from unknown samples must be compared to some known concentration or standard. For this purpose, a **standard curve** is prepared from known concentrations of protein. The ideal protein sample should be identical to the protein under investigation. However, since this is not always possible, a protein such as bovine serum albumin (BSA) may be substituted. The protein is accurately weighed, put into solution, diluted appropriately, and the various dilutions assayed. Figure 6.1 gives an example of a standard curve that can be obtained using the Lowry method with BSA as the standard protein. Samples were prepared containing from 1 to 250 µg of protein per ml, and readings were taken at $A_{500}$. Remember that the relationship found in the standard curve applies only for the specific conditions under which the standard curve was developed.

To save time, this exercise can be performed in groups of four students. Two students can prepare the standard curve while the other two prepare the precipitates.

## MATERIALS

(Per group)

> BSA
> 13 × 100-mm tubes
> Lowry reagent (see appendix for preparation)
> Folin-Ciocalteu phenol reagent
> 1-ml pipettes
> Spectrophotometer
> Precipitates from exercise 5
> Saline
> Coomassie Brilliant Blue reagent

## PROCEDURE

### Preparation of a Standard Curve

**Lowry method**
1. To prepare a standard curve with BSA, make dilutions of BSA in saline to give 10, 25, 50, 100, 250, 500 and 1,000 µg of BSA per ml. Keep the **total volume** in each tube at 1.0 ml. BSA will go into solution best if the BSA is added to saline and set aside (at 4° C) without shaking. Prepare one tube with no BSA and use

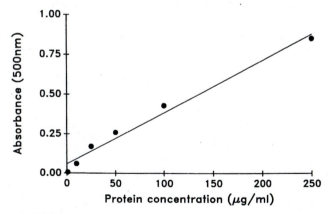

**FIGURE 6.1**
A protein standard curve. The curve obtained by the student may differ from the one shown here depending upon the protein used as the standard.

as a blank. Treat this tube with reagents exactly as the other tubes are treated.

2. Add 1 ml of Lowry reagent to each tube. Mix, and allow the tubes to incubate at room temperature for 30 min. See the appendix for information about the preparation of Lowry reagent.

3. After the incubation period, add 0.5 ml of Folin-Ciocalteu phenol reagent to each tube and mix immediately. Incubate the tubes at room temperature for 30 min to allow color development.

4. Although readings may be taken at any wavelength from $A_{500}$ to $A_{750}$, calibrate a spectrophotometer at $A_{500}$ with the **blank tube** and take readings at this wavelength.

5. Plot the absorbance versus the protein concentrations of each dilution of BSA.

### Bradford method

1. Complete step 1 as outlined above.

2. Add 1 ml of Coomassie Brilliant Blue reagent to each tube and mix with a vortex mixer. Allow color to develop for at least 2 min.

3. Determine the $A_{595}$ and make the standard curve by plotting absorbance for each known concentration of protein as in step 5 above.

## Preparation of the Precipitation Curve

1. Perform the Lowry or Bradford procedure on the precipitates saved from step 8 of exercise 5 as follows.

2. Drain all the excess water from the sediments in the four tubes. It is critical that no part of the sediment from any tube is lost.

3. Dissolve the precipitate in each of the four tubes in 1.0 ml of saline, then add the appropriate reagents as outlined above. Mix well and incubate.

4. Standardize a spectrophotometer with the blank which is reagent without protein. Measure absorbance of each sample at the appropriate wavelength.

5. With these readings determine the protein concentrations of the sediments from the standard curve. Draw a precipitation curve. Determine the zone of antigen and antibody excess. Determine the equivalence point.

## DISCUSSION

These methods also require patience and good laboratory skills. Follow carefully procedures to obtain accurate and quantitative results.

Many investigators prepare a standard curve based on a nitrogen assay of the protein studied. The Kjeldahl method is frequently used for this purpose. Additionally, the standard curve is prepared from a protein with the same composition as the protein under investigation, because each protein gives a color that is significantly different from others.

It will become obvious from the student's standard curve that protein concentration and absorbance show a linear relationship over a very small range of protein concentrations. Linearity is lost somewhere around 200 mg of protein/ml of sample and, therefore, samples should contain less than that for accurate readings. Samples that are too concentrated to be estimated from the standard curve should be diluted and assayed again.

## SELECTED REFERENCES

Bradford, M. M. 1976. A rapid and sensitive method for the quantitation of microgram quantities of protein utilizing the principle of protein dye binding. *Anal. Biochem.* 72:248.

Lowry, O. H., N. J. Rosenbrough, A. L. Farr, and R. J. Randall. 1951. Protein measurement with Folin phenol reagent. *J. Biol. Chem.* 193:256.

# Agglutination

## INTRODUCTION

Agglutination results when homologous antibody reacts with **particulate antigen,** principally cells such as bacteria, yeasts or erythrocytes. With appropriate conditions, such a reaction produces visible results because of the formation of a lattice. The lattice is composed of antibodies bridged between antigens (figure 7.1). A large number of epitopes are present on the surface of a cell. Divalent or multivalent antibodies specific for these react with them, and cross-linking results. IgM and, to a lesser extent, IgG are good agglutinating antibodies.

Agglutination reactions are useful in typing blood, determining antibody titers of sera, and identifying bacterial cells. This highly sensitive method has been adapted for many clinical procedures. Agglutination is also convenient and fast.

One important aspect of agglutination is the ability of **soluble** antigens to be attached to particulate matter (carriers). When these antigens come in contact with specific antibodies, an agglutination reaction results. The agglutination results from the antibody reacting with the attached antigen, not with the carrier. Red blood cells, polystyrene latex (0.8 μ in diameter), collodion, and bentonite (hydrated aluminum silicate) serve as examples of routinely used antigen carriers.

**Hemagglutination** implies agglutination of erythrocytes by antibodies. Antibodies may be directed to specific blood group antigens such as the major antigens (A and B) or to minor antigens and are useful in typing blood. In this case the antigens are known as isoantigens and the test for these is known as **isohemagglutination. Passive agglutination** results from reactions of antibody with soluble antigens coupled to carriers, particularly latex beads, and **passive hemagglutination** results from the reaction of antibodies with soluble antigens that have been coupled to erythrocytes. Agglutination of the latex beads or red cells simply indicates an antigen-antibody reaction, and the beads or cells play only a passive role.

## MATERIALS

A. Blood typing (Per pair)

Lancets
Alcohol swabs
Microscope slides
Anti-A typing serum
Anti-B typing serum
Anti-Rh (anti-D) typing serum
Adhesive bandages

B. Bacterial agglutination (Per pair)

a. *Slide test*

Serum specimen
Agglutination microscope slides
0.2-ml pipettes
*Salmonella* H and O antiserum (prepared commercially)
*Salmonella* H and O antigen (prepared commercially)
Saline
Wooden applicators

b. *Tube test*

11 clean, sterile 13 × 100-mm test tubes
Saline
1 sterile 16 × 150-mm test tube
1.0-ml pipettes
0.2-ml pipettes
*Salmonella* antiserum and antigen as above
50° C water bath

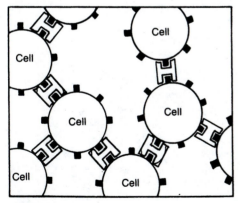

**FIGURE 7.1**
Antigen and antibody react to produce an aggregation of cells held together by antibodies. The aggregation is called a lattice. The antibodies are shown reacting with the antigenic determinant sites on the cells.

## Blood Grouping by Agglutination

The presence of isoantigens must be determined prior to blood transfusion to eliminate the possibility of hemoglobinurea or other serious transfusion reactions. These reactions generally occur when recipient antibodies react with transferred erythrocytes. Such a reaction in the vascular system of the recipient may result in death.

Typing of erythrocytes for ABO type involves having a blood specimen and two isoantibodies, anti-A and anti-B. A drop of blood to be tested is placed on a slide and mixed with a drop of anti-A. Another drop of blood is mixed with anti-B. Within a few minutes the agglutination reaction is complete if homologous antigens and antibodies are present. If the A antigen is present, red blood cells will be ag-

glutinated by anti-A. If B antigens are present, red blood cells will be agglutinated by anti-B. Some erythrocytes have both A and B and will be agglutinated by anti-A and anti-B. If neither antigen is present, no agglutination will occur with either antiserum (figure 7.2). In addition, some individuals have another important red blood cell antigen called the **Rh antigen.** Also important in transfusion reactions, it can be detected with anti-Rh antiserum. A drop containing Rh positive erythrocytes and a drop of anti-Rh antiserum mixed on a **warm slide** will result in agglutination.

Humans have a number of different blood group systems, but they are not all equally important in transfusion reactions. The severity of a transfusion reaction depends upon the antibody class and concentration.

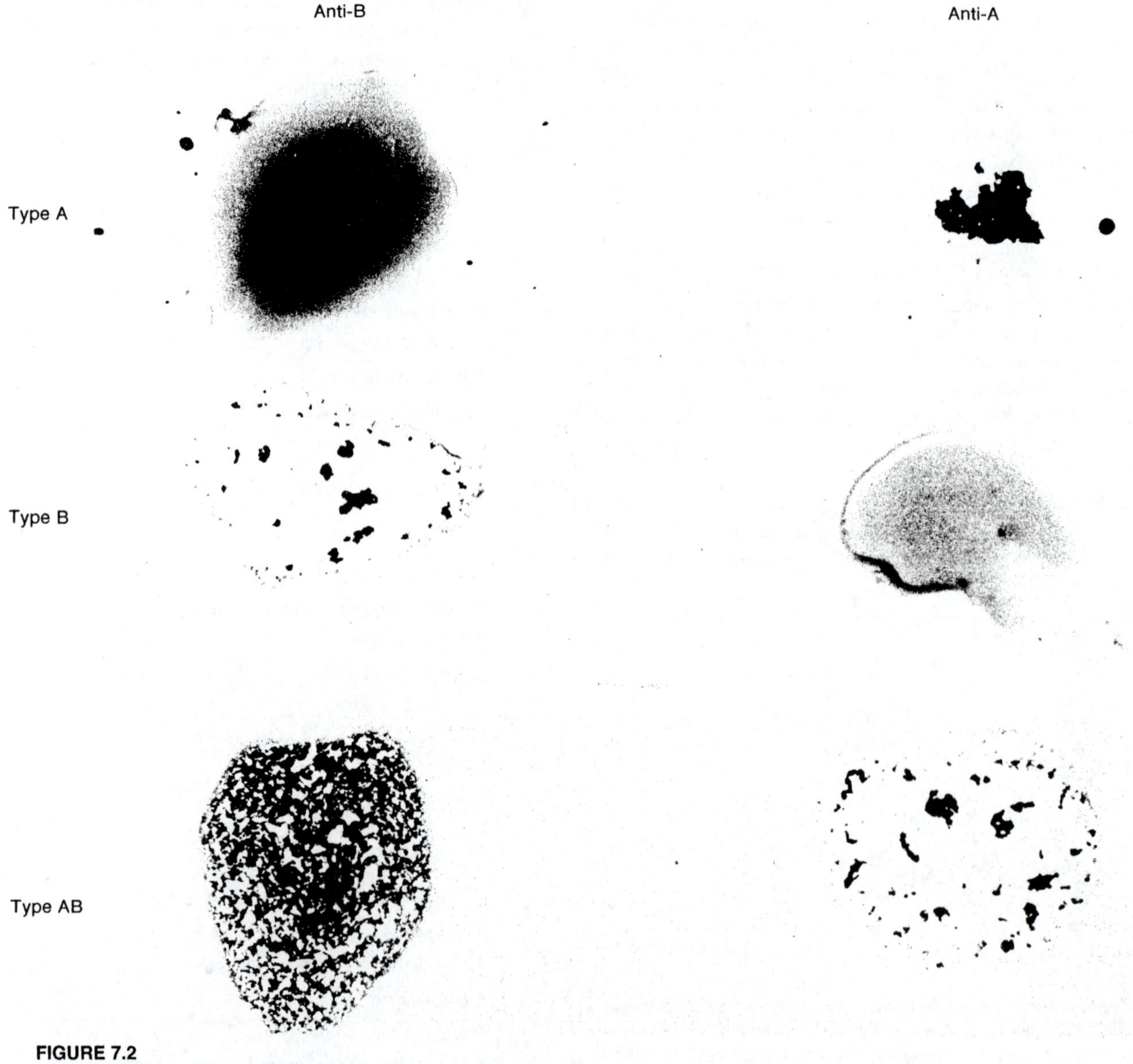

**FIGURE 7.2**

The agglutination (clumping) of red blood cells occurs when red blood cells with A type antigens are mixed with anti-A antibodies and when cells with B type antigens are mixed with anti-B antibodies.

© Stuart I. Fox

## Bacterial Agglutination

When patients are infected with certain bacteria (particularly those that possess antigens that cause persistent fever), the individual responds by producing antibodies that are referred to as agglutinating antibodies. The antigens are called febrile antigens and are characteristic of such microorganisms as *Salmonella, Francisella, Leptospira* and some *Rickettsiae.* Agglutination tests allow one to detect and quantify antibodies in serum of infected individuals. The individual, however, may not respond immunologically to microbial antigens and, therefore, a negative test does not necessarily preclude infection.

In addition to detecting antibodies in patient's serum, agglutination tests can identify microorganisms. The microbiologist may isolate the causative agent and want to confirm the identification. Agglutination tests are designed not as substitutes for conventional identification methods, but rather as adjunct procedures. The original test, called the **Widal agglutination reaction,** was designed as a laboratory test to aid in the diagnosis of typhoid fever. It was done on a microscope slide and yielded quick results. A rising titer of specific agglutinating antibodies over time was accepted as evidence of infection. The procedure has not changed much since the original method was described.

Although commercially prepared antigens and hyperimmune antisera (produced in goats) are available, the student may want to prepare them. An **H antigen** suspension can be prepared by inoculating an infusion broth with the bacterium and incubating for 24 hr at 37° C. After incubation, add an equal volume of 0.6% formol-saline and incubate for 1 hr. Centrifuge the cells and dilute with saline to $1 \times 10^8$ cells/ml. An **O antigen** suspension can be prepared by boiling a cell suspension for 1 hr at 100° C. Pellet the cells and resuspend with saline to $1 \times 10^8$ cells/ml. These antigen suspensions may be diluted before use. An antiserum specific for these antigens can be prepared as outlined in exercise 1.

Two tests are normally used. The **slide test** will be completed first. It is a rapid and widely used test that is not quantitative but does provide an indication that antibodies are present in the patient's serum. Serum is diluted so that false negative results are not obtained due to a prozone (presence of too many antibodies) effect.

The second test is run only when positive results are obtained from a slide test. Designed to confirm the original findings, the **tube test** is quantitative and involves the serial dilution of patient's serum. Diluted serum is placed in tubes, and a constant amount of the appropriate antigen added to each. The agglutination pattern is observed and recorded. Controls are simultaneously run in both tests. The agglutination test can be run on several sera at once using a microtiter method so that smaller amounts of serum are used.

In this exercise, both tests use serum with antibodies to *Salmonella.* The three recognized species of this genus include *S. cholersuis, S. typhi,* and *S. enteritidis. S. enteritidis* contains more than 100 serotypes with common antigens.

## PROCEDURE

### ABO Blood Typing

1. Secure clean microscope slides.
2. Divide a slide in half with a marking pencil. One end will be used to test for A antigen, the other for B antigen. Label the slide appropriately.
3. Using procedures described in exercise 3, prick your finger and place a drop of blood on each half of the slide.
4. Quickly add a drop of anti-A typing serum to one drop of blood and a drop of anti-B typing serum to the other.
5. Mix each with a clean wooden applicator or rotate the slide on a serological rotating device to enhance the reaction.
6. Observe for agglutination within 2 min.

### Rh Blood Typing

1. Follow the procedure given above for obtaining a drop of blood and place it on a microscope slide. Label appropriately.
2. Quickly add a drop of anti-Rh (anti-D) antiserum.
3. Mix as above, or rotate or place on a serological rotator and read the results within 2 min. (Some serologists prefer to warm the slide for optimum results.)

### Slide Test

1. Using procedures for the collection of blood previously described, obtain a serum specimen (test serum) that is suspected of containing antibodies to *Salmonella* or use the test specimen provided. Also use control sera that do or do not contain antibodies for a double check. These are referred to as positive and negative controls, respectively.
2. Label clean microscope slides or use special hollow-ground slides (depression slides). Slides that are blackened on the opposite side are easier to read. Five marked areas on a slide or five depressions will be sufficient for test serum, and the same number will be necessary for positive control serum. Provide an additional 2 areas or depressions for negative control serum.
3. Carefully pipette 0.08, 0.04, 0.02, 0.01 and 0.005 ml of the test serum into the appropriate areas or

depressions with a 0.2 ml serological pipette. These volumes are to be read as 1:20, 1:40, 1:80, 1:160 and 1:320 dilutions, respectively. Why?

4. At the same time, pipette the same quantities of positive control serum into similar areas or wells.
5. Prepare a negative control (saline) with both the test serum and the positive control serum by placing a drop of saline onto the slide.
6. Dispense one drop of appropriate antigen (undiluted) onto each serum dilution as well as onto negative controls.
7. Immediately stir each mixture with a clean wooden applicator and then carefully rotate for approximately 1 min. A mechanical rotator may be used.
8. Read and record the results as follows.

A **positive slide test** results in a fine flocculation or granulation that is visible to the naked eye. To read the results it is necessary to determine the **degree of agglutination** and is recorded as 4+, 3+, 2+, 1+, +−, or − where:

4+ is complete agglutination of cells
3+ is 75% agglutination of cells
2+ is 50% agglutination of cells
1+ is 25% agglutination of cells
+− is trace agglutination of cells
− is no agglutination of cells

## Tube Test

1. Prepare a $5 \times 10^7$ cells/ml suspension in saline of the bacteria to be used in the test. Get 10 Kahn tubes ($13 \times 100$ mm) for each serum to be tested and place in a rack. Have sufficient saline and a 50° C water bath ready to use.
2. Pipette 0.9 ml of saline into the first tube of each series and 0.5 ml into each of the remaining tubes.
3. Pipette 0.1 ml of the serum to be tested into the first tube of the series. Use a 0.2 ml pipette to increase accuracy. Mix.
4. Pipette 0.5 ml from tube 1 into tube 2 in each series. Use a 1.0 ml pipette. Mix.
5. Pipette 0.5 ml from tube 2 into tube 3 in each series. Use a 1.0 ml pipette. Mix.
6. Continue this procedure until the dilution procedure is complete through tube 10. Discard 0.5 ml from tube 10. The dilution procedure just completed has produced the following dilutions of serum; 1:10, 1:20, 1:40, 1:80, 1:160, 1:320, 1:640, 1:1,280, 1:2,560, and 1:5,120. Explain.
7. Prepare an **antigen control** by adding 0.5 ml of saline to another tube.
8. Pipette 0.5 ml of the antigen from step 1 above into all tubes. Mix the contents of all tubes thoroughly on a vortex mixer.
9. Incubate in a temperature-controlled water bath. The O antigens should be incubated at 50° C for 18 hr and the H antigens at the same temperature for 1 hr.
10. Read and record the results as follows:

*Salmonella* sp. contain two basic antigens. The O or somatic antigen is heat-stable and, when involved in an antigen-antibody reaction, produces a granular agglutination that will settle to the bottom of the tube. The H or flagellar antigen produces a fluffy agglutination that may be easily broken up. The titer of a tube test is read by determining the **degree of agglutination** and is recorded as 4+, 3+, 2+, 1+ or − as follows:

4+ is complete agglutination with clear supernatant
3+ is 75% agglutination with slightly cloudy supernatant
2+ is 50% agglutination with moderately cloudy supernatant
1+ is 25% agglutination with cloudy supernatant
− is no agglutination

## DISCUSSION

These tests provide evidence that the patient has an infection caused by a particular *Salmonella* strain. The tests are also useful for typing *Salmonella*.

The slide test is usually performed with an O polyvalent *Salmonella* antiserum. A positive serum should then be tested again with individual O group antisera. When the group determination has been made, the isolate should be tested with polyvalent H antisera. When making a conclusion about the presence of disease from the agglutination tests, an agglutination titer of more than 1:50 indicates infection. This determination must be made during the illness and is not valid if the patient was vaccinated within the past 2 years.

The concept of a **control** should be clear from this exercise. Subsequent exercises will have controls included as **standards for comparison.** Controls are untreated systems that are included as checks so that the effects of treatments can be determined.

## SELECTED REFERENCES

Bryant, N. J. 1982. *An introduction to immunohematology.* 2d ed. Philadelphia, PA: W. B. Saunders Co.

Delaat, A. N. C. 1976. *Primer of serology.* New York, NY: Harper and Row.

Friedman, H., T. J. Linna, and J. E. Prier, eds. 1979. *Immunoserology in the diagnosis of infectious diseases.* Baltimore, MD: University Park Press.

# Commercial Agglutination Tests

## INTRODUCTION

Agglutination is an in vitro test to detect the presence of agglutinating antibodies in serum. This exercise explores the use of several **agglutination tests** used in **clinical immunology.** These have been prepared commercially for use in detecting antibodies in patients' serum or to detect the presence of antibodies or antigens in other body fluids.

Since most antigens used in the following tests are soluble, they have been **adsorbed onto inert carriers** such as polystyrene (latex), erythrocytes, or charcoal to enhance the sensitivity of the test. Carriers that have been coated with antigen are used in constant amounts and are agglutinated with serial dilutions of antiserum.

The tests used in this exercise have been purchased from different manufacturers, and the directions that follow are consistent with the manufacturer's instructions. Most kits include both positive and negative controls to be used for comparison to reactions observed for patients' specimens. Include controls in all tests. Bring all sera and other reagents to room temperature before use. All sera used in tests of this kind must be handled with care and considered to be **potentially hazardous** due to the possibility of contamination with infectious agents.

## MATERIALS

Each diagnostic kit includes the following items:

Test slides
Applicators
Positive control
Negative control

### A. Pregnancy test

Student or other test urine specimen
Urine specimen containers
Antigen reagent (HCG-latex)
Antiserum reagent (anti-HCG)
Droppers
Pipettes
Applicator sticks
Black glass slide

### B. Streptococcal grouping

Culture of different species of *Streptococcus* on blood agar plates
Clean 13 × 100-mm test tubes
Streptococcal grouping kit with extraction fluid and latex grouping sera
Pipettes (0.5 ml and Pasteur)
37° C water bath

### C. SLE latex test

Student or other test serum specimen
Glass agglutination slides
SLE reagent
Positive control serum
Negative control serum
Pipettes

### D. Antistreptolysin O latex test

Student or other test serum specimen
Clean 13 × 100-mm test tubes
Saline
5-ml pipettes
ASO latex reagent
ASO positive control serum
ASO negative control serum
Glass agglutination slide
Pipettes

### E. C-Reactive protein latex test

Student or other test serum specimen
Clean 13 × 100-mm test tubes
1.0-ml pipettes
CRP latex reagent
CRP positive control serum
CRP negative control serum
Glass agglutination slide

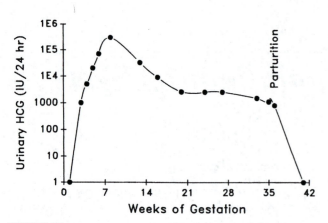

**FIGURE 8.1**
Human chorionic gonadotropin (HCG) is produced during pregnancy and can be used as an indicator of pregnancy.

### F. Rapid plasma reagin card test

Student or other test serum specimen

RPR antigen suspension

RPR card test agglutination cards

Pipettes

Control sera

Antigen dispensing vial

### G. Hemagglutination test for infectious mononucleosis

Student or other test serum specimen

Clean black glass agglutination slide

Latex reagent

Positive control serum

Negative control serum

Pipettes

Stirrers

## Pregnancy Test

This test, used to determine pregnancy, takes advantage of the fact that pregnant women excrete a placental hormone called **human chorionic gonadotropin** (HCG) in urine. Figure 8.1 indicates the approximate amounts of HCG normally present in urine over the 36-week gestation period. An agglutination reaction detects the presence of the hormone, and a positive test indicates pregnancy. This test provides a good example of **hemagglutination inhibition.**

Since HCG is a soluble antigen, it is possible to produce precipitating antibodies to it by injecting HCG into a rabbit. The antibodies to HCG are collected, purified and used as the test reagent. The other reagent used is the hormone, HCG, attached to spherical latex particles. When the hormone is mixed with the antibody-latex complex, it produces a visible agglutination reaction.

To run the test, mix urine with rabbit anti-HCG. If HCG is present, a specific antigen-antibody reaction will result, but it is not visible. Anti-HCG is used up in the reaction. When HCG-coated latex is added, there will be no residual antibody to form a visible agglutination reaction with the HCG-coated latex. The antibodies have essentially been neutralized by the HCG in the urine. No agglutination (hemagglutination inhibition) is a **positive test** since the hormone is present in the patient's urine. If HCG is not present, anti-HCG will be available to react with the HCG-coated latex particles, and a visible agglutination does occur. This is indicative of a **negative test.**

The pregnancy test is performed as a macroscopic slide agglutination test. Patient's urine is mixed with anti-HCG on a slide. HCG-coated latex particles are then added and mixed, and after a suitable incubation period, the result is read. This sensitive test will detect as little as 1.5 International Units (IU) of HCG per ml of urine which are levels found very early in pregnancy.

## PROCEDURE (ROCHE PREGNOSIS®, FISHER DIAGNOSTICS, ORANGEBURG, NY)

1. Urine should be collected in a clean container. Morning urine provides maximum sensitivity.
2. Obtain a clean black glass slide that has been washed in a mild detergent and thoroughly rinsed.
3. Add one drop of patient's urine to the microscope slide using the disposable pipette included in the test kit. Add another drop of positive control urine to another slide.
4. Add one drop of anti-HCG to each drop of urine using the dropper provided. Mix. Do not cross-contaminate either the patient's specimen or the control.
5. Before using, shake the HCG latex reagent. Add one drop of this reagent to each mixture on the slides with the dropper provided. Mix.
6. Rotate by hand, mix with an applicator stick, or place on a serological rotator for 2 min.
7. Read the results immediately. For best results read agglutination under direct light.
8. A positive test has no agglutination; a negative test has agglutination.

## Streptococcal Grouping

This test provides a rapid agglutination test for the detection and identification of the **Group A streptococci** described by Lancefield. Most clinical isolates belong to either group A, B, C, D, F or G.

As with many bacteria, members of the genus *Streptococcus* have specific antigens that are actually part of the cell wall structure. These antigens are usually carbohydrates

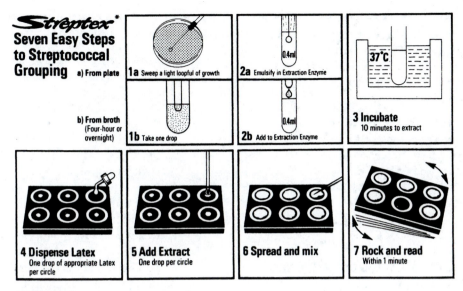

**FIGURE 8.2**
The steps used to group streptococci based on the Streptex™ method.
Courtesy Murex Diagnostics, Inc.

and can be enzymatically extracted to produce a soluble antigen extract.

The literature describes several extraction procedures, and many of these tests utilize a proteolytic enzymatic extraction procedure. Group-specific antibodies can be raised to these soluble antigens and coated onto the surface of latex beads. When an enzyme extract of the streptococcal antigens in question is mixed with latex beads coated with the appropriate group-specific antibody, the latex beads will agglutinate. Agglutination indicates a positive test for a specific Lancefield group of streptococci.

## PROCEDURE (MUREX DIAGNOSTICS, INC. STREPTEX,™ NORCROSS, GA)

1. Figure 8.2 outlines the procedure for this test. Colonies of bacteria suspected of being *Streptococcus* should be well-isolated colonies on blood agar. **Note:** precautions used in handling pathogenic microorganisms should be practiced throughout this test.
2. Prepare a light suspension of the bacterium to be tested in 0.4 ml of extraction fluid in a clean 13 × 100 mm tube. It may be necessary to use 4 or 5 colonies.
3. Incubate the bacterial suspension in a 37° C water bath for 10 min. This produces the antigen extract.
4. Carefully mix each of the latex suspensions provided in the kit to ensure complete mixing.
5. Pipette a single drop of each latex suspension onto a different site on the clean disposable reaction card which is provided.

6. Carefully dispense a drop of the antigen extract onto a drop of each latex suspension. Label appropriately.
7. Mix each with a clean wooden applicator.
8. Rotate the slide manually until positive agglutination of at least **one antigen extract and latex suspension occurs.** Rotate for a maximum of 1 min. A strong agglutination of only one of the antigen extracts is sufficient to record a positive identification.
9. Read and record the results.

## SLE Test

This latex agglutination test identifies antibodies that react with nucleoprotein substances found associated with the autoimmune disease, systemic lupus erythematosis (SLE). SLE is a connective tissue disease that occurs primarily in young females. Many organ systems may be involved, but damage to the kidneys presents the greatest clinical problem.

Antibodies (antinuclear antibodies) found in patient's serum are directed against deoxyribonucleohistones (DNP) and occur in about 90% of patients with the disease. A positive agglutination slide test is based on the fact that antinuclear antibodies will react with stabilized animal erythrocytes that have been coated with DNP, producing a visible agglutination. The following test is a rapid slide agglutination test, but a titration procedure can be devised to produce a quantitative result.

**Table 8.1** Enzymes Produced by the Group A Streptococci. Assays for Presence of These Enzymes Are Useful for Grouping These Bacteria.

| Enzyme | Function |
|---|---|
| Streptolysin O | Lyse erythrocytes and other cells |
| DNase | Depolymerize host DNA |
| Hyaluronidase | Break down host connective tissue |
| Streptokinase | Dissolve blood clots |
| NADase | Break NAD down to nicotinamide and ADP |
| Proteinase | Hydrolyze proteins |

## PROCEDURE (BAXTER IMMUNOSCAN™ SLE TEST, MCGRAW PARK, IL)

1. Obtain a clean glass agglutination slide that has been washed in a mild detergent. Have test sera available.
2. Pipette 1 drop (40 μl) of the test serum and controls onto the glass slide.
3. Gently shake the SLE reagent to suspend the erythrocytes and pipette one drop onto the test sera.
4. Mix each with a different clean applicator.
5. Rotate the slide manually for no more than 1 min. Place on a flat surface and do not disturb for 1 min.
6. Observe for agglutination in indirect light and record the results. Agglutination indicates the presence of antinuclear antibodies.

## Antistreptolysin O Test

Group A β-hemolytic streptococci produces several extracellular enzymes which act as toxins (table 8.1). Notable among these is a substance known as streptolysin O, a hemolysin. This substance, produced during the infectious process, induces an antibody response. The antibodies, known as antistreptolysin O (ASO), indicate diseases such as rheumatic fever and glomerulonephritis. Actually, two distinct hemolysins are produced. Streptolysin O is rapidly oxidized in the presence of oxygen, but the other is oxygen-stable and is called streptolysin S.

This test uses latex beads coated with streptolysin O, which serves as the antigen. Patient's serum containing antibodies is added and after a suitable incubation period, agglutination is recorded. The test may simply provide a qualitative determination, but by making appropriate dilutions of serum, a quantitative titration may be obtained. The following test provides a qualitative determination of antibodies in serum.

## PROCEDURE (BAXTER IMMUNOSCAN™ ASO TEST, MCGRAW PARK, IL)

1. Have all reagents ready to use. Gently mix the ASO latex reagent. Obtain a clean agglutination slide.
2. In a 13 × 100-mm tube, mix 0.5 ml of saline and 0.1 ml of the test serum specimen. This produces a 1:6 dilution of serum. Mix.
3. Pipette a 0.05 ml of the diluted serum onto the agglutination slide.
4. Using a pipette, dispense one drop of the ASO latex reagent onto the serum.
5. Mix with a clean stirrer.
6. Gently rotate for 3 min. Observe for agglutination in direct light. Repeat with the positive and negative controls.
7. Record results. Agglutination indicates a positive test.

## C-Reactive Protein Test

Some time ago it was discovered that a particular protein substance could be found in the serum of patients with various disease states. The protein appeared during the acute phase and was designated **C-Reactive Protein** (CRP). It is now known that CRP, an abnormal glycoprotein, appears in the serum of patients with diseases that are characterized by **acute inflammation,** such as rheumatoid arthritis and rheumatic fever.

Since CRP is a protein, antibodies can be raised against it, and the antibodies can be used in immunoprecipitation techniques to detect the presence of CRP. To enhance sensitivity of antigen detection, the antibody can be coated onto the surface of latex particles and mixed with patient's serum. Agglutination is noted. When CRP is present in serum, the agglutination reaction that results indicates an inflammatory process within the patient and serves as an indicator of disease.

## PROCEDURE (BAXTER IMMUNOSCAN™ CRP TEST, MCGRAW PARK, IL)

1. Prepare a clean glass agglutination slide by washing with a mild detergent. Secure a serum specimen, warm all reagents to room temperature, and mix all reagents.
2. Pipette 0.05 ml of the test serum onto the glass slide.
3. Add one drop of CRP latex reagent to the serum and mix.
4. Manually rotate the mixture for 3 min and read under direct light. Repeat the procedure for positive and negative controls.

5. Observe the slide under reflected light for evidence of latex agglutination. Record the results. Agglutination indicates a positive test.

## Rapid Plasma Reagin Card Test

The **Rapid Plasma Reagin Card Test,** a quick and sensitive method to determine the presence of antibody to the syphilis spirochete, is thus useful in diagnosis of syphilis. It is a variation of the Venereal Disease Research Laboratory (VDRL) test and was originally designed as a field test using either plasma or serum from the patient. This greatly simplifies the test. The antibody, traditionally called **reagin,** is produced during an infection caused by *Treponema pallidum.*

This test differs from other agglutination tests described in that the antigen suspension contains **charcoal particles.** In addition, the antigen is a cardiolipin preparation, and, instead of a glass agglutination slide, the test uses a disposable, plastic-coated cardboard agglutination card. Cardiolipin is a heterophile antigen, a substance from one organism that elicits the formation of antibodies that are capable of reacting with tissues from other organisms.

As in other agglutination tests of this nature, the antigen contained on charcoal particles is mixed with patient's serum (or plasma for this test). Agglutination indicates a positive test.

### PROCEDURE (BAXTER IMMUNOSCAN™ RPR CARD TEST, MCGRAW PARK, IL)

1. Have the card, reagents and test serum ready to use. Be sure to resuspend the antigen by gently shaking the vial before use.
2. Deliver 1 drop (0.05 ml) of the specimen onto an appropriate area of the card. Label accordingly. (See manufacturer's instructions for the exact procedure.)
3. Add 1 drop of antigen from the dispensing vial onto the serum specimen. **Do not mix.**
4. Place the card on a mechanical rotator and mix for 8 min at approximately 100 rpm. Repeat the procedure for the control sera.
5. After taking the card from the rotator, gently rotate by hand as agglutination is observed. Use direct lighting.
6. The results are reported as follows:
   a. Reactive—black clumping of charcoal particles.
   b. Nonreactive—a gray, nonhomogenous suspension of charcoal particles.

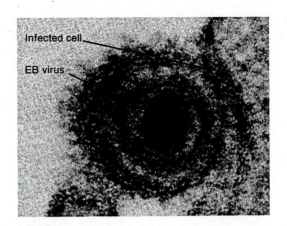

**FIGURE 8.3**
An electron photomicrograph of the Epstein-Barr virus (EBV) infecting a human cell.
© Dr. Jack Griffith

**Table 8.2** A Partial List of Viruses That Produce Human Non-Respiratory Disease.

| Virus | Viral Disease |
|---|---|
| Coxsackievirus A | Meningitis (aseptic) |
| Coxsackievirus B | Myocarditis |
| Cytomegalovirus (CMV) | Cytomegalovirus inclusion disease |
| Epstein-Barr (EB) | Infectious mononucleosis |
| Herpes simplex | Encephalitis |

## Test for Infectious Mononucleosis

The first report of antibodies in serum that could agglutinate sheep cells was reported by Paul and Bunnell, and the test they developed is known as the Paul-Bunnell test. This was the first test to detect **heterophile antibodies** specific for infectious mononucleosis, a disease with a low mortality that is assumed to be caused by a herpes-like agent known as the Epstein-Barr virus (EBV) (figure 8.3). The disease is characterized by a short febrile period with cervical lymph node enlargement.

Other **rapid diagnostic methods** for a variety of viral agents include: (1) cytological studies, (2) viral antigen detection, (3) electron microscopy examinations, and (4) serology determinations. Viruses listed in table 8.2 all produce non-respiratory disease and may be identified using one or more of these methods. However, all but EBV can be routinely isolated in the clinical virology laboratory.

The test used in this exercise detects heterophile antibodies using a mononucleosis antigen obtained from bovine red cell membranes attached to latex particles. When a patient's serum is added, a typical agglutination reaction indicates infectious mononucleosis.

## PROCEDURE (WAMPOLE LABORATORIES® MONO-LATEX® SLIDE TEST, CRANBURY, NJ)

1. Have a serum specimen available and use a clean black glass agglutination slide.
2. Place a drop of patient's serum on the slide. Do likewise with a positive and negative control.
3. Add one drop of test reagent to each. Mix separately.
4. Rotate gently for 2 min and then read agglutination immediately using direct lighting.
5. Record results. Agglutination indicates a positive result.

## DISCUSSION

One benefit of the use of immunological techniques in the clinical laboratory has been to decrease the time necessary for a confirmed diagnosis of disease. The **rapidity and specificity** imparted by the antigen-antibody reaction can verify other phenomena such as nucleic acid hybridization (e.g., DNA probes). In this case biotin-avidin-enzyme conjugates attach to single-stranded nucleic acid probes to detect nucleic acids of several viruses and bacteria in clinical specimens.

With any diagnostic procedure, **false positives** do occur. Therefore, students should incorporate appropriate controls into the test. Manufacturers usually provide advice to the user when there are questions about specificity of the test. The tests suggested for use in this exercise only represent samples of those that are available. The instructor should refer to the insert included with each kit for additional instructions.

## SELECTED REFERENCES

Albertini, A., and R. Ekins, eds. 1981. *Monoclonal antibodies and developments in immunoassay.* Amsterdam: Elsevier/North-Holland, Biomedical Press.

Bryant, N. J. 1992. *Laboratory immunology and serology.* 3d ed. Philadelphia, PA: W. B. Saunders Co.

Friedman, H., T. J. Linna, and J. E. Prier. 1979. *Immunoserology in the diagnosis of infectious disease.* Baltimore, MD: University Park Press.

Galvin, J. P. 1985. Particle-enhanced immunoassays. In *Manual of Clinical Laboratory Immunology.* 3d ed. Edited by Rose, N. R., and Friedman, H. Washington, DC: American Society for Microbiology.

Henry, J. B. 1979. Infectious mononucleosis. In Todd-Stanford-Davidsohn, *Clinical diagnosis and management by laboratory methods.* 16th ed., chap. 3:1049. Edited by Nelson, D. A., et al. Philadelphia, PA: W. B. Saunders Co.

Kohler, G., and C. Milstein. 1975. Continuous cultures of fused cells secreting antibody of predefined specificity. *Nature.* 256:495.

Larsen, S. A., V. Pope, and T. T. Quan. 1992. *Immunologic methods for the diagnosis of spirochetal diseases.* In *Manual of Clinical Laboratory Immunology.* 4th ed. Edited by Rose, N. R., E. C. Macario, J. L. Fahey, H. Friedman, and G. M. Penn. Washington, DC: American Society for Microbiology.

Perryman, M., S. Larsen, E. Hambie, D. Pettit, R. Mullally, and W. Whittington. 1982. Evaluation of a new rapid plasma reagin card test as a screening test for syphilis. *J. Clin. Microbiol.* 16:286.

# Electrophoresis

## INTRODUCTION

This exercise demonstrates the movement of particles in an electric field by a process known as **electrophoresis.** The sample used is serum, and results in the separation, identification, and, if desired, the estimation of the amounts of protein in fractions of the serum sample. Particles to be separated must be in solution and possess an overall positive or negative charge. Several factors influence the rate of movement, but the important ones include: (1) the chemical nature of the particles, (2) the buffer, and (3) the electric current. Related factors include the molecular weight of the particles, the pH, ionic strength, and viscosity of the buffer, and the magnitude of the charge.

The particle will migrate in an electric field to the pole of opposite charge. Protein antigens and antibodies contain both positive and negative charges, but the pH of the buffer solution dictates the net charge of the molecule. At the appropriate pH, the protein will be at the isoelectric point where there is no charge and thus no migration. At an acid pH an amino acid will be a cation, and at an alkaline pH it will be an anion.

An electrophoretic apparatus (see figure 9.1) consists of two chambers each containing an electrode. The chambers are filled with a buffer that serves as the electrolyte. The sample is applied or spotted onto a wetted piece of cellulose acetate paper (or other appropriate solid support) which is stretched between the chambers with the ends dipped in the buffer. The electrodes are connected to a high voltage source, and a direct current is applied.

A tracing dye may be added to the sample to be electrophoresed so that the progress of migration of the components can be monitored. After an appropriate time period, the paper is removed, dried, and stained for observation of results.

After staining the strip, the student should see a result similar to that shown in figure 9.2. Since the intensity of staining relates to the amount of protein present, it is possible to estimate (or quantitate) serum protein components. The student can quickly determine relative amounts of proteins in serum by scanning the stained, cleared, and dried strips with a recording densitometer. Figure 9.3 shows a typical curve obtained by this method. However, in the exercise described below, students will estimate protein quantity by a spectrophotometric method.

Electrophoresis of serum is used in the clinical laboratory as a **diagnostic tool.** For example, hypogammaglobulinemia and analbuminemia give characteristic electrophoretic patterns. In hypogammaglobulinemia the quantity of the gamma globulin fraction appears to be very low as indicated by the degree of staining, and the rest of the pattern remains relatively stable. Table 9.1 lists changes in protein fractions associated with certain diseases. Table 9.2 presents the average normal values for serum protein.

The procedure described in this exercise involves separation of serum proteins. However, the electrophoretic method can be used for the separation of other substances such as lipoproteins, isoenzymes, and hemoglobulin.

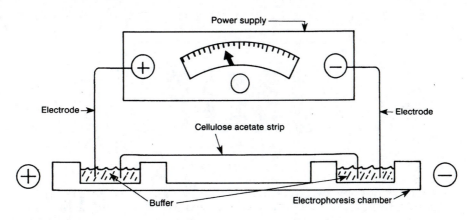

**FIGURE 9.1**
An electrophoresis apparatus. A cellulose acetate strip with a sample applied to it is placed on the instrument with one end in buffer with the negative electrode and the other end in buffer with the positive electrode. Current is applied and separation proceeds.

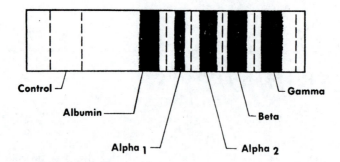

**FIGURE 9.2**

Cellulose acetate electrophoretic pattern of normal human serum. The direction of travel in this figure is to the left (anode). Fractions can be further studied by eluting components from the strip. For this the strips should be cut along the dotted line. One strip containing no protein should serve as the control.

Reproduced with permission from John D. Bauer, *Clinical Laboratory Methods*, ed. 9, 1982. St. Louis, 1982, The C. V. Mosby Co.

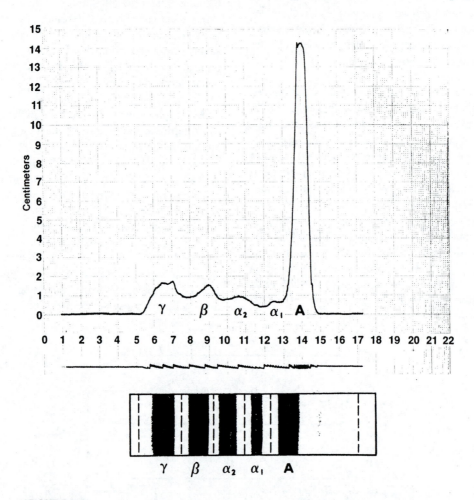

**FIGURE 9.3**

Results obtained by scanning a cellulose acetate strip with a densitometer. A, albumin; alpha$_1$ and alpha$_2$, alpha-globulins; beta, beta-globulins; gamma, gamma-globulins.

Reproduced with permission from John D. Bauer, *Clinical Laboratory Methods*, ed. 9, 1982. St. Louis, 1982, The C. V. Mosby Co.

**Table 9.1**  Changes in Electrophoresis Protein Fractions Associated with Diseases

| | Total protein | Albumin | α₁-Globulin | α₂-Globulin | β-Globulin | γ-Globulin |
|---|---|---|---|---|---|---|
| Acute infection | | D | | I | | |
| Asthma and other allergies with poor response to therapy | | D | | I | | D |
| Carcinomatosis | | D | I | I | | |
| Chronic infection | | D | | | | I |
| Cryoglobulinemia | | | | | | I |
| Diabetes mellitus | | D | I | I | | |
| Glomerulonephritis | D | D | I | | | |
| Hepatic cirrhosis | D | D | | | | I |
| Hepatitis, viral | | D | D | D | I | I |
| Hodgkin's disease | D | D | | I | | I |
| Leukemia, myelogenous | | D | | | | I |
| Lupus erythematosus | | D | | I | | I |
| Lymphoma and lymphocytic leukemia | D | D | | | | D |
| Macroglobulinemia | I | D | | | I | I |
| Myeloma | I | D | | | | I |
| Myasthenia | | D | | | | I |
| Myxedema | | D | | I | | I |
| Nephrosis (highest A₂ elevation) | D | D | | I | | D |
| Rheumatic fever | | D | | I | | |
| Rheumatoid arthritis | | D | | I | | I |
| Sarcoidosis | I | D | | I | I | I |
| Scleroderma | D | D | D | D | D | D |
| Ulcerative colitis and other exudative enteropathies | D | D | I | I | D | D |

I = increase; D = decrease.
Source: Bauer, *Clinical Laboratory Methods,* ed. 9, The C. V. Mosby Co., 1982, p. 500, table 21−4.

## MATERIALS

(Per group of 4)

Barbital buffer (pH 8.6)

Cellulose acetate electrophoresis strips

Ponceau S protein staining solution

Wash solution (5% acetic acid)

Electrophoretic unit

Staining troughs

Wash troughs

Student or other test serum samples

Sample application (spotting) apparatus or micropipette

Spectrophotometer

Razor blades

13 × 100-mm test tubes

Clearing solvent (1 part formic acid and 9 parts dimethylsulfoxide)

Spectrophotometric cuvettes

Pipettes

**Table 9.2**  The Normal Range of Serum Protein Concentrations, Determined by Cellulose Acetate Electrophoresis

| Fraction | Concentration in serum g/dl | Percent of total protein |
|---|---|---|
| Albumin | 3.7–5.7 | 54–74 |
| Globulin | | |
| α₁ | 0.1–0.3 | 1.1–4.2 |
| α₂ | 0.4–1.0 | 4.6–13.0 |
| β | 0.5–1.0 | 7.3–13.5 |
| γ | 0.5–1.5 | 8.1–19.9 |
| TOTAL PROTEIN | 6.5–8.2 | 100 |

Source: Bauer, *Clinical Laboratory Methods,* ed. 9, The C. V. Mosby Co., 1982, p. 499, table 21–3.

Forceps
Blotting paper
Power supply
37° C incubator

## PROCEDURE

1. This exercise produces electrophoretic separation of normal serum on cellulose acetate strips. Use standard barbital buffer at pH 8.6 to 8.8. See the appendix for the formulation. High-resolution buffers designed and already prepared especially for electrophoresis can be purchased.
2. Set up a standard electrophoretic apparatus. Follow the manufacturer's and instructor's directions for proper use and read the safety instructions in exercise 13.
3. Fill the two chambers with electrophoresis buffer.
4. Place a strip of cellulose acetate in the buffer in one chamber and allow it to remain until saturated with buffer. Use forceps instead of your fingers to handle the strip.
5. Remove the strip and blot off the excess buffer. Immediately apply 2 μl of the serum sample to the cellulose acetate strip. Apply the sample at an area on the strip that will allow movement of serum components in either direction. Use a micropipette or a special applicator designed for this purpose. Carefully follow additional instructions presented for application. Specimen application is a critical part of this exercise, and improper application will lead to poor results.
6. Place the strips across the support on the electrophoresis instrument with the ends of the strips dipping into the appropriate buffer chamber.
7. Adjust the power supply to 10 to 30 mA at a potential of 200 to 300 volts and run for approximately 60 min.
8. Remove the strips after 60 min or when it is determined appropriate and place into Ponceau S solution in a staining trough and stain the strip for 5 min. See the appendix for the preparation of the stain.
9. Wash in 5% acetic acid in wash troughs until all of the background stain is removed.

10. Observe the results at this point but continue with the following procedure for estimating the amount of protein in each serum fraction.
11. Make certain that the cellulose acetate strip stained in step 8 above is free of any excess stain. Dry it at 37° C.
12. Using a single-edge razor blade, cut the strip into sections with each containing one obvious band of protein. Use figure 9.2 as a guide. Place each section into a separate 13 × 100-mm test tube.
13. Add **exactly 5 ml** of clearing solvent to each tube. The solvent will dissolve the cellulose acetate.
14. With the wavelength set at $A_{520}$, standardize a spectrophotometer with clearing solvent alone.
15. Finally, determine the absorbance for each tube from step 13 and analyze the results.
16. The absorbance for each sample will be proportional to the amount of protein in that fraction. How would you determine the fractional percent of a particular sample? Prepare a bar graph to indicate fractional percentages.

## DISCUSSION

The buffered solutions used provide good resolution. More complex buffers may not necessarily provide greater resolution and barbital works well at the desired pH. However, store this buffer at cold-room temperatures to preserve it.

Good resolution depends upon the method and care used to apply the sample. To be able to quantitate the separated components, samples must be applied to avoid trailing that produces bands that are not easily separated for quantitation. Quantitation is easier when the electrophoretic steps are done properly. Likewise, the length of time used for electrophoresis must be sufficient to allow good separation.

## SELECTED REFERENCES

Andrews, A. J. 1981. *Electrophoresis.* New York, NY: Oxford University Press.

Bollag, D. M., and S. J. Elelstein. 1991. *Protein methods.* New York, NY: Wiley-Liss.

Turgeon, M. L. 1990. *Immunology and serology in laboratory medicine.* St. Louis, MO: C. V. Mosby Co.

# Gel Diffusion

## INTRODUCTION

The **gel diffusion** technique, modified many times since the original description by Ouchterlony in 1948, seems to have an infinite number of variations. However, they all allow the student to determine the purity, homogeneity and number of antigen-antibody groups present. Most modifications combine: (1) diffusion and (2) precipitation. The reaction involves diffusion of antigen and antibody in a semisolid medium to a point in the medium where optimum concentration of each is reached. At this point precipitation occurs, and results in a visible **band of precipitate.** A commonly used method (Ouchterlony) involves **double diffusion** where both reactants diffuse toward one another. When they have met at the point of optimal concentration ratio of antigen to antibody, a band of clearly visible precipitate forms. The band indicates that antibody has precipitated antigen.

A macro- or micro- method may be used. The difference involves the amount of reactants and, therefore, the distance of migration necessary to produce visible results. Agar may be poured into a Petri dish or onto a microscope slide and allowed to harden. Appropriate wells are punched in the agar, and reactants are carefully placed into separate wells. Upon incubation, diffusion occurs, producing precipitation bands.

Use an agar of a refined or purified grade, so that impurities will not interfere with the reaction. It should be prepared in buffer at pH 8.4 to 8.6 to allow for maximum reaction. When the diffusion agar has solidified, wells are punched according to a predetermined pattern. One useful pattern consists of a **central well with circumferential wells** equal distances from the central well. After addition of antigen and antibody to the appropriate wells, plates are incubated in a humidity chamber to prevent drying and observed periodically until precipitation is evident. Incubation temperature can vary. Some prefer to incubate at 4° C, but this temperature increases reaction time.

A major advantage of the Ouchterlony method (or a modification of it) occurs because it can detect more than one antigen-antibody system in a mixture. When an antiserum containing a number of different antibodies diffuses toward another well containing a mixture of antigens, several bands will form, each indicative of a specific antigen-antibody system. The method is extremely sensitive and able to detect a few milligrams of antigen and antibody. It will also detect similarities of components (figure 10.1).

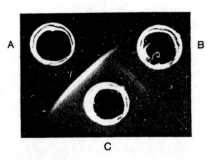

**FIGURE 10.1**
Immunoprecipitation showing partial identity of antigens, specifically streptolysin O and *Listeria monocytogenes* hemolysin. A = purified streptolysin O; B = purified hemolysin. C = undiluted anti-streptolysin O.
Source: In *Infection and Immunity* 55(7): 1643, figure 2.

The second part of this exercise is a single radial immunodiffusion (SRID) technique important in determining the amount of antigen in solution. The technique was originally developed by Fahey and McKelvey and later refined by Mancini and others.

The method can be used routinely in the clinical immunology laboratory to determine serum immunoglobulin concentration, as well as complement, C-reactive protein, alpha-fetoprotein, or transferrin. It has important applications in the research laboratory as well. SRID is basically a **single gel diffusion technique.** Antibody is incorporated into purified agar, and when antigen diffuses into the agar and reacts with antibody, a precipitate forms. If the antibody is in the agar in a uniform concentration, a quantitative determination of antigen can be made by measuring the diameter of the area of precipitation.

Basically, the technique involves cutting a cylindrical well and filling it with antigen. The well must be prepared carefully because nicks at the edges of the well cause distortions in the precipitation ring and give erroneous determinations. In addition, the antigen must be applied to the well so that there is no spilling outside the well. The test is incubated a suitable period of time to allow an endpoint to be reached.

In the early stages of diffusion, antigen reacts with antibody where there is antigen excess, and as a result, forms soluble complexes. As diffusion continues, a state of optimum concentration of both reactants is reached, and a visible precipitation ring is formed. The more antigen present, the greater the diameter of the precipitation ring (figure 10.2).

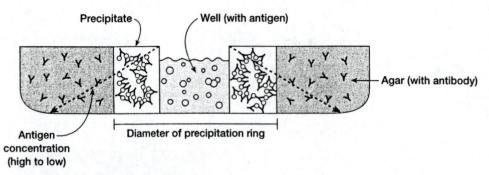

**FIGURE 10.2**
A side view of the mechanism of precipitation formation in agar. After addition of antigen to the well, diffusion occurs radially into the agar containing antibody. The concentration of antigen is always highest near the well and lower further from the well. The precipitate forms in the area of optimum concentration of antigen and antibody.

The results are read by measuring the diameter of the ring, and comparing this reading to the size of precipitation rings produced by **known concentrations** of antigen. These are used to plot a reference curve (figure 10.3), and concentrations of test sera are determined from the reference curve. Preparation of the curve is explained in detail later.

Radial immunodiffusion plates are commercially available for quantitation of antibodies such as IgG, IgA or IgM in patient's serum or plasma. In these tests the patient's antibody serves as the test antigen. Kits are supplied with standard concentrations of immunoglobulin for the preparation of reference curves. However, plates can be prepared to determine the concentration of any soluble antigen to which a specific antibody is available.

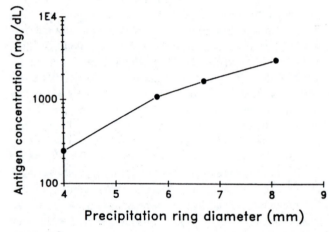

**FIGURE 10.3**
A reference curve for determining the concentration of antigen from the diameter of the precipitation ring.

## MATERIALS

A. Double diffusion
   (Per pair)

   1-ml pipettes
   1 tube BSA (1%)
   5 13 × 100-mm test tubes
   2 sterile 15 × 60-mm Petri dishes
   1 125-ml flask
   1 tube anti-BSA
   Purified agar
   Saline
   Capillary pipettes
   Human antiserum
   Human serum
   Barbital buffer (see the appendix for preparation)
   Choose 2 of the following:
      Bovine serum
      Equine serum
      Murine serum
      Rabbit serum

B. Single diffusion
   (Per pair)

   Standard controls for IgG and IgM
   Student or test serum specimens
   IgG SRID plates
   IgM SRID plates
   Microliter pipettes
   Measuring ruler
   Semi-log graph paper

## PROCEDURE

### Double Diffusion

1. The first part utilizes a one-antigen system of bovine serum albumin (BSA). The antibody is anti-BSA. The second part, a one-antigen system, uses human serum and antihuman serum, but the antiserum will also be tested against

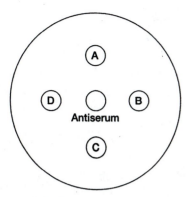

**FIGURE 10.4**
A well pattern for the Ouchterlony technique. Place a 15 × 60-mm Petri dish filled with immunodiffusion agar over the pattern and punch wells 5 to 6-mm apart, according to the pattern. Remove the plugs and fill the wells with antigen or antibody.

serum from other species. The instructor may substitute other antigen-antibody systems.

2. Prepare 25 ml of agar by adding 0.25 g of purified agar to 25 ml of barbital buffer. This is double-diffusion agar. See the appendix for the preparation of the buffer. Pour 12 ml of hot agar into each of two, 15 × 60-mm Petri dishes and allow to harden. Some investigators add Trypan Blue to enhance the visualization of precipitation bands.

3. Prepare doubling dilutions of BSA (1%) from 1:200 to 1:1,600 with saline as the diluent. This will produce 4 dilutions to add to wells.

4. Place the pattern in figure 10.4 under the Petri dishes containing hardened agar and punch holes with the propipette end of a capillary pipette or other appropriate tool according to the well pattern. Suction out the plug. The well should have **smooth edges** for best results.

5. Fill the center well of one Petri dish with anti-BSA (approximately 0.05 ml). Add 0.05 ml of each dilution of antigen from step 3 to other wells. Be careful not to let the reactants overflow the wells.

6. To the center well of the other plate, add approximately 0.05 ml of antihuman serum. Fill one peripheral well with 0.05 ml of human serum, one with saline (control), and the other two with either equine serum, bovine serum, murine serum, or rabbit serum.

7. Cover and incubate the plates at 4° C for up to 4 days. Examine them frequently.

8. Record and interpret the results. Explain why the anti-BSA-BSA system produced precipitation bands at different distances from the center well.

## Single Diffusion

1. This procedure quantitates serum antibodies. Several kits are available for this procedure, and the instructions that follow are useful for most, but are specifically intended for the NOR-Partigen™ kit made by Behring Diagnostics (Westwood, MA). Manufacturer's directions and specifications should be **strictly followed.** Methods include reading results at 18, 24, 48 or up to 80 hr for some classes of antibodies.

2. Radial immunodiffusion plates with an **18-hr overnight readout** will be used in this experiment.

3. Select wells for the calibration of a **reference curve** for IgG and IgM. Deliver 5 μl of each of the standard control sera provided to separate wells. Your instructor will tell you the concentrations of the standards.

4. Other wells should be filled with 5 μl of undiluted **test samples.** Fill the wells carefully. Do not allow the sample to spill out and take care not to damage the wells.

5. Place a cover over the plates, place in a moist chamber to prevent drying, and incubate at room temperature.

6. Measure the diameters of the precipitation rings at endpoint (18 hr exactly). Measurements should be made to the nearest 0.1 mm.

7. Plot the **diameter of the rings** obtained from the standard control sera on the x axis and the concentration of each control serum (mg/dL) on the y axis of semi-log graph paper. Use this as the reference curve from which values for unknown sera can be determined. For example, a zone of precipitate with a diameter of 6 mm is produced from 1350 mg/dL of IgG in a patient's serum as determined from the reference curve in figure 10.3. Keep in mind that a separate curve must be prepared from standards for determination of each antibody class.

8. Measure the diameter of the precipitation rings of the unknown sera and determine the antigen (antibody) concentration from the reference curve as described in step 7.

## DISCUSSION

The Ouchterlony method is important because it allows one to determine **relationships between antigens.** For example, antigens in adjacent wells in a plate produce precipitation bands that overlap if the antigens are not identical. If they are **identical,** the two bands form a continuous line, and if there is **partial identity** of the antigens, a spur forms, as shown in figure 10.1.

The double diffusion procedures provided here present the student with two results. The first measures antibody concentration. The other answers questions about similarities of serum proteins between species. The method is sensitive to temperature and the concentration of components.

Some individuals may want to use International Units as a means for expressing concentration of antibodies derived by the single-diffusion technique. These units have been standardized by the World Health Organization, which provides international reference standards for comparison purposes. Conversion factors can be calculated by calibrating standards provided in kits with reference standards provided by the World Health Organization.

Problems associated with the SRID procedure can include distorted rings if the sample wells have not been properly prepared or if the wells are not filled properly. The plates provide the best results if they are incubated at appropriate temperatures and not allowed to dry out. Patient samples are undesirable if antibodies have been affected by such things as proteolytic enzymes.

If done properly, the **expected normal human adult** serum antibody values are:

800 to 1800 mg/dL for IgG
60 to 250 mg/dL for IgM

## SELECTED REFERENCES

Fahey, J. L., and E. M. McKelvey. 1965. Quantitative determinations of serum immunoglobulins in antibody agar plates. *J. Immunol.* 94:84.

Mancini, G., A. O. Carbonara, and J. F. Heremans. 1965. Immunochemical quantitation of antigens by single radial immunodiffusion. *Immunochem.* 2:234.

Weir, D. M., L. A. Herzenberg, C. Blackwell, and Leonore A. Herzenberg. 1986. *Handbook of experimental immunology.* 4th ed. Boston, MA: Blackwell Scientific.

# Antibody Detection, Isolation and Analysis

This section of the laboratory manual introduces the student to some of the newer techniques, developed within the past few years, that apply in both the research and clinical immunology laboratory. The idea for inclusion of this series came from hearing a presentation at a national meeting of the American Society for Microbiology by Thomas A. Brawner, Ph.D., Professor, Biology Department, Carthage College, Kenosha, WI. Dr. Brawner indicated that he has excellent success with these experiments in his immunology course and encouraged their use. They readily apply to the laboratory study of immunology and are relatively easy for beginning immunology students to perform. The exercises in this section, written by Dr. Brawner, are included with minor modifications.

These exercises are intended to be performed sequentially. The first procedure (exercise 11) allows the student to become familiar with the ELISA procedure. An antigen (rabbit IgG) is attached to microtiter wells and a peroxidase conjugate (anti-rabbit IgG) is used to assay for the antigen. Dilution of antigen and antibody provides a means to titer the antiserum and will be useful in exercises that follow. Additionally, sensitivity and specificity of the method becomes obvious when students analyze results.

Once the ELISA has been mastered, the student begins a series of three experiments that involve the isolation and analysis of a class of antibody molecules. The ELISA procedure provides a means to **detect** purified antibody. Affinity chromatography (exercise 12) is the method used to **purify** rabbit IgG. The Bio-Rad Laboratories (Hercules, CA) procedure is suggested for this and other procedures that follow, but several other available methods may be easily substituted. Once rabbit serum passes through an affinity column and eluent is monitored with a UV absorbance monitor, fractions are analyzed for IgG using the ELISA procedure.

The next procedure (exercise 13) uses SDS-PAGE to **separate** the proteins in eluents collected in the previous exercise. Students will cast gels, run them, and analyze the result. Although the experiment appears complicated at first glance, the instructor and students will find the directions easy to follow and results worth the effort. The introduction stresses safety considerations and a results section notes applications of the method.

Finally, exercise 14 introduces immunoblotting, also called Western blotting, as a means of **detecting** and **identifying** a specific protein. The proteins in the gels produced in exercise 13 are blotted onto a nitrocellulose membrane and specific components (rabbit IgG) identified with anti-rabbit IgG peroxidase conjugate. Since prestained molecular weight standards are run concurrently, students will be able to prepare a molecular weight standard curve and make conclusions about the molecular weight of the rabbit IgG.

Student interpretation of results of this combination of exercises, along with exercise 1, introduces them to **scientific writing.** Having produced a specific antibody in a rabbit in exercise 1, students can detect it with ELISA, isolate it with affinity chromatography, and analyze and identify it with SDS-PAGE and Western blotting. The results of these rather sophisticated experiments provide data that can be presented in an acceptable format—appropriate for a paper submitted to a scientific journal for review. Other students may serve as a review panel that makes suggestions to students submitting the paper and may accept or reject it. This requires students to be serious about these laboratory procedures and critically analyze the results. It provides important writing experience, and the required survey of the literature creates familiarity with the current journals.

*Figure III presents the approximate instructor preparation time and student laboratory time necessary for successful completion of exercises 11 through 14.*

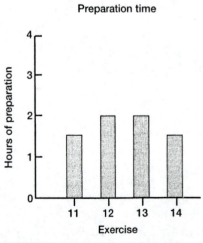

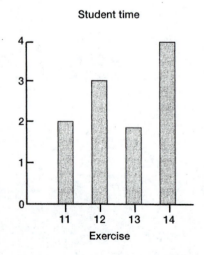

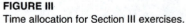

**FIGURE III**
Time allocation for Section III exercises.

# 11

# *Enzyme-Linked Immunosorbent Assay (ELISA or EIA)*

## INTRODUCTION

Several different ELISA (Enzyme-Linked Immunosorbent Assay) systems can detect antibodies or soluble antigens. In all of these systems one reactant is bound to a solid phase and the other, in turn, binds to the first. The method used in this exercise, a **direct ELISA,** will detect soluble antigen. Often this method is used to screen for antigens because it provides a rapid and sensitive assay with few steps. Figure 11.1 outlines the procedure.

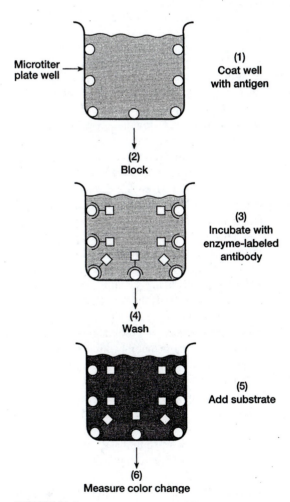

**FIGURE 11.1**
The direct ELISA procedure for antigen detection.

Other ELISA methods include the indirect method, which is normally used for antibody screening; the highly sensitive antibody-sandwich method, which is used for antigen screening; the double antibody-sandwich method is used for antibody screening; and, finally, other methods screen for antigens associated with tissues and cells.

In the direct method described in this exercise, students will detect and quantitate soluble antigens. It is a serial dilution procedure used to determine optimal concentrations of antigen and antibody for later use. The procedure has been called a **criss-cross serial dilution analysis.** Plastic **microtiter plate wells** are coated with soluble antigen which may be available only in microgram amounts. After incubation with a blocking buffer to reduce nonspecific reactions, a specific **antibody-enzyme conjugate** is added to the antigen-coated wells and an antigen-antibody reaction results. The unbound antibody is washed from the wells and the enzyme substrate is added. Since the substrate is chromogenic, it produces a colored product as the bound enzyme conjugate hydrolyzes the substrate. The color of the product, detected visually or measured with a spectrophotometer, depends upon the enzyme and substrate selected. The amount of color produced is proportional to the amount of antigen originally bound to the microtiter well (figure 11.2).

Benefits of the method include sensitivity and quantitation, and it requires very little equipment. The procedure may be designed for more elaborate equipment such as automatic diluters and microtiter plate readers. The necessary biologicals are readily available and relatively inexpensive.

In the following procedure, IgG in rabbit serum serves as the antigen and will be attached to the solid phase. Anti-rabbit IgG with a peroxidase conjugate will be used to assay for IgG. The substrate, *o*-phenylenediamine dihydrochloride, is a chromogen widely used in ELISA procedures. It produces a soluble end product that is orange-brown in color and can be easily read spectrophotometrically.

## MATERIALS

96-well microtiter plates (flat bottom)
Micropipette with disposable tips
Adhesive covers

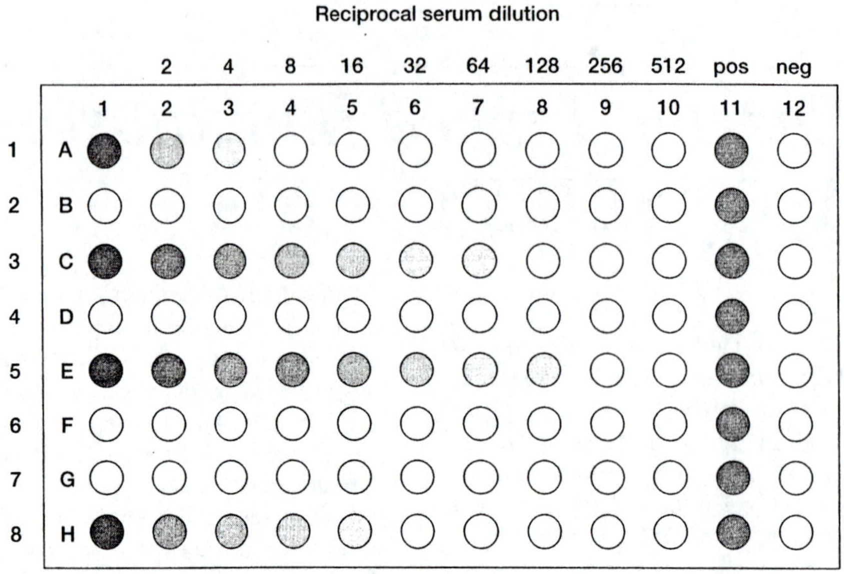

Reciprocal serum dilution

**FIGURE 11.2**
Results of ELISA procedure in a 96-well microtiter plate. Different test sera were added to wells in column 1 and diluted through column 10. Positive and negative controls are in columns 11 and 12, respectively. The plate is an example of assessment of antibody in various test sera by measuring the absorbance of the colored end product.

Antigen (rabbit serum, available commercially or from exercise 1)

Coating buffer (See the appendix for the formulation of buffers)

Diluting buffer

Wash buffer

Saline

Anti-rabbit IgG peroxidase conjugate

Substrate (*o*-phenylenediamine dihydrochloride prepared according to manufacturer's instructions)

Spectrophotometer (or microtiter plate reader)

## PROCEDURE

1. Note the design of the 96-well microtiter plate, with its 12 columns and 8 rows of wells. The columns are usually designated 1 through 12 and the rows are designated A through H. The wells will hold small amounts of reagents and are specifically designed to bind antigens or antibodies.

2. Your instructor will demonstrate the use of **micropipettes.** Some deliver a liquid to a single well while others deliver to eight wells at the same time (multichannel pipette). All have disposable tips. Some investigators prefer to use automatic pipetters/diluters, but whichever micropipette is chosen, you will use the micropipette to add, dilute, and mix reagents from well to well.

3. Carefully fill columns 2 through 12 of the microtiter plate with 50 μl of the coating buffer.

4. Place 100 μl of rabbit serum (antigen) in each well of column 1. Using the following protocol, serially dilute the antigen in coating buffer that was added to the wells in step 2. Starting in row A, column 1 of the microtiter plate and continuing through row A, column 11, make two-fold dilutions by taking 50 μl from well 1 and transferring it to well 2. Mix by pipetting up and down 4 or 5 times. Repeat this procedure through column 11. Remove 50 μl from column 11. Do not add antigen to column 12 because this will serve as the blank. Continue the above procedure for rows B through H. An alternative method uses an automatic pipetter/diluter that mixes and delivers the desired amount. The student should note that this dilution series results in a range of twofold dilutions of rabbit serum (containing IgG) from undiluted in column 1 through 1:1,024 in column 11. Explain.

5. Seal the plate with an adhesive cover and incubate overnight at 4° C. Alternatively, the plates can be wrapped in plastic wrap to seal. After coating is complete, plates can be stored for long periods of time.

6. After overnight incubation, carefully remove the seal. Pour off the antigen solution by turning the plate over and shaking the liquid from the wells into the sink.

7. Fill each well with 200 μl of diluting buffer. Some procedures refer to diluting buffer as blocking buffer because it inhibits additional binding of reactants to the well. Replace with a new piece of adhesive tape.
8. Incubate the microtiter plates at room temperature for 45 min.
9. At the end of the incubation period, remove the diluting buffer by pouring it into the sink. Add 50 μl of diluting buffer to all wells of row B through row H. This begins the steps used to dilute the antibody conjugate.
10. Add 100 μl of enzyme-labelled antibody conjugate (anti-rabbit IgG peroxidase conjugate) diluted in diluting buffer to all wells in row A. A recommended starting dilution of conjugate is 1:100. Serially dilute conjugate from row A to row H using the pipetting and diluting procedure described in step 4. The final volume of the conjugate in each well should be 50 μl. The final dilution from row A to row H should be 1:100 to 1:12,800. Be sure to use a new tip when changing columns.
11. Cover the plate with adhesive tape or plastic seal and incubate for 45 min at 37° C.
12. At the end of the incubation period, remove the tape and pour and then shake the reagents into the sink.
13. Carefully wash the plates four times using wash buffer. The wash may be accomplished by filling all wells from a wash bottle containing wash buffer and then inverting the plate over the sink. Shake to remove excess wash buffer. Following the last wash, invert the plate over a paper towel and pat the plate on the paper towel to dry.
14. Add 50 μl of the peroxidase substrate-buffer solution (o-phenylenediamine dihydrochloride) to which $H_2O_2$ has been added just prior to use to each well (See appendix for procedure) and incubate at room temperature in the dark for 15 to 30 min. After the first 10 min of incubation, check each 5 min for color development. Stop the incubation when no color is seen in the control wells (column 12) and color appears in rows on the left side of the plate.
15. At the end of the incubation period, add 200 μl of 1N HCl to each well to stop the enzyme reaction.
16. Quickly, pipette the mixture from each well of the microtiter plate into a 13 × 100 mm tube, add 3 ml of distilled water, and mix. Transfer this to a spectrophotometer tube.
17. Read the intensity of the color reaction in each tube in a spectrophotometer at $A_{495}$. Record the data so that the technique may be used to determine the sensitivity of each antibody dilution. Be sure to consider the results obtained with the appropriate control.

## DISCUSSION

The sensitivity of an ELISA depends on many factors, including the assay configuration (format), class of immunoglobulin used as the detecting antibody, purity of the detecting antibody, and concentration of the antibody-conjugate. The selection of an appropriate antibody-conjugate concentration depends on the final use of the assay. Increased concentration of antibody-conjugate may result in greater sensitivity while sacrificing the ability to discriminate between antigens (specificity). In addition, an increase in the amount of antibody-conjugate in the reaction mixture may have a detrimental effect on the background seen in the control wells.

Explain the reason for the dilution pattern used in the microtiter plate. Would you expect to see the same results if a higher concentration of enzyme conjugate were used? What caused the decrease in color (signal) seen? The controls (column 12) should be colorless or have only a slight color. What could be the reason for an intense color present in any of these wells? What effect would the presence of color in wells found in column 12 have on your interpretations of the results?

## SELECTED REFERENCES

Cattaneo, C., K. Gelsthorpe, and R. J. Sokol. 1993. Blood residues on stone tools: Indoor and outdoor experiments. *World Archaeol.* 348:552.

Engvall, E., and P. Perlman. 1971. Enzyme-linked immunosorbent assay (ELISA): Quantitative assay of immunoglobulin G. *Immunochem.* 8:871.

Hornbeck, P. 1991. Assays for antibody production. In *Current protocols in immunology.* Edited by J. E. Coligan, A. M. Kruisbeek, D. H. Margulies, E. M. Shevach, and W. Strober. pp. 2.1.1–2.3.4. New York, NY: Greene Publishing and Wiley-Interscience.

Kurstak, E. 1986. *Enzyme immunodiagnosis.* San Diego, CA: Academic Press.

Zaaijer, H. L., and E. Altena. 1992. Early detection of antibodies to HIV–1 by third-generation assays. *Lancet.* 340:770.

# 12

# Affinity Chromatography

## INTRODUCTION

A number of procedures exist for the concentration and purification of antibodies. These include ammonium sulfate precipitation, size exclusion chromatography (see exercise 20), affinity chromatography, and ion-exchange chromatography. Each method has advantages and produces antibodies of high purity. The choice of a method depends upon the preferences of the investigator. **Affinity chromatography** methods especially apply when speed and reasonably high purity are desired.

In this procedure students will purify IgG molecules from rabbit serum using **Protein A linked to agarose.** Protein A, isolated from *Staphylococcus aureus* or produced by recombinant DNA technology, has the ability to bind to the Fc portion of immunoglobulins from a variety of animal species including the rabbit. It has the unique property of binding selectively to IgG. When bound to agarose beads to form a solid phase, it can be packed into a column and samples selectively eluted to remove IgG (figure 12.1). The technique has been used extensively for the purification of **monoclonal antibodies.**

With appropriate conditions, a high percentage of IgG in a variety of animal sera can be separated from other components. A column connected to a fraction collector provides a means of collecting appropriate samples that have been detected by a flow-through UV monitor. Figure 20.2 shows an appropriate arrangement for instrumentation used in this experiment.

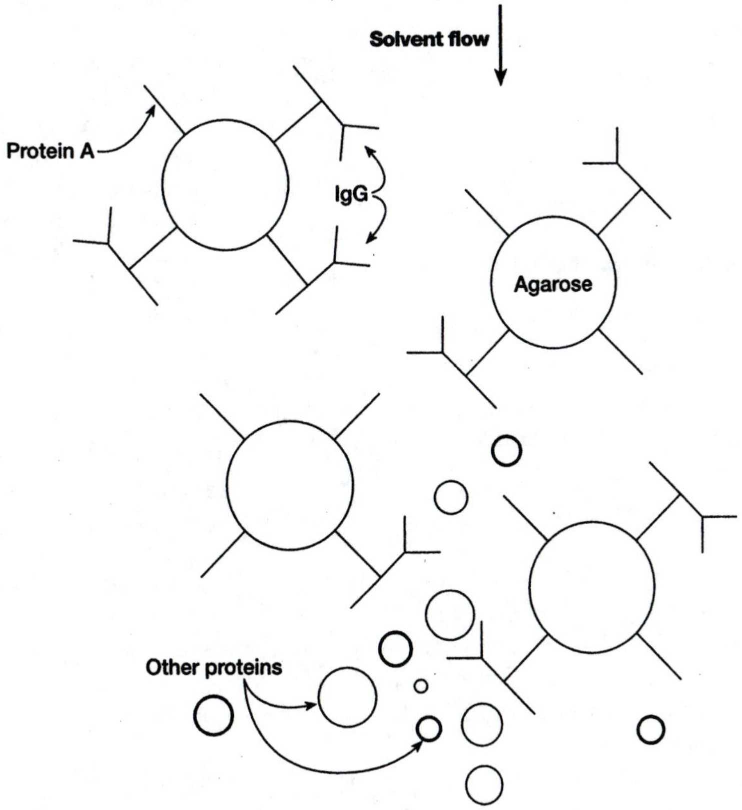

**FIGURE 12.1**
As solvent containing IgG passes through a column containing Protein A bound to agarose, IgG selectively binds to the Protein A.

The procedure described in this exercise uses materials purchased from Bio-Rad Laboratories and utilizes the Affi-Gel® Protein A MAPS® II kit. The kit includes most of the necessary materials. Following the separation of rabbit serum, fractions will be examined using the ELISA procedure performed in exercise 11. The ELISA procedure, with minor modifications, allows the student, to determine if IgG has been successfully separated from other components.

## MATERIALS

Chromatography

> Affi-Gel® Protein A agarose in 0.05 M sodium phosphate, pH 7.5
>
> Binding buffer, pH 9.0 (see appendix A for the formulation of buffers)
>
> Elution buffer, pH 3.0
>
> Regeneration buffer
>
> Chromatography column ($1 \times 10$ cm)
>
> Rabbit serum
>
> Pump (optional)
>
> Flow-through UV monitor
>
> Fraction collector
>
> 1 M Tris HCl, pH 9.0

ELISA

> 96-well microtiter plates (flat bottom)
>
> Adhesive covers
>
> Coating buffer
>
> Diluting buffer
>
> Wash buffer
>
> Saline
>
> Anti-rabbit IgG peroxidase conjugate (diluted by the instructor)
>
> Substrate (*o*-phenylenediamine dihydrochloride, prepared according to manufacturer's instructions)
>
> Micropipette with disposable tips
>
> Spectrophotometer (or microtiter plate reader)

## PROCEDURE

### Packing the Column

1. Secure a $1 \times 10$ cm column to a column rack. Use spring-loaded clips or other devices to hold the column in place. Tubing should be attached to the top and bottom and the column attached to suggested instrumentation.

2. The instructor will determine whether to use a peristaltic pump or gravity feed materials into the column. If a pump is used, a flow rate of 1 to 5 ml/min generally proves adequate for separation as outlined below. Open the top of the column and add 1 ml of binding buffer. Tap the column to remove bubbles.

3. Add 3 ml of Protein A agarose (gel) with a pipette. It has been previously determined that 1 ml of Protein A agarose will bind 6 to 8 mg protein/ml gel and, therefore, 3 ml of gel should provide separation of ample IgG for further study.

4. Equilibrate the column. This can be accomplished by running 5 bed volumes of binding buffer through the column. The effluent should have a pH of 9.0, which is the pH of the binding buffer. At the same time, the eluate should have an $A_{280}$ at baseline on the absorbance monitor or when checked with a spectrophotometer.

### Sample Application

5. Dilute rabbit serum 1:4 in binding buffer and carefully layer 2 ml onto the top of the Protein A agarose bed. Overloading can be determined, if desired, by testing for antibody activity of unbound fraction.

6. Carefully allow binding buffer to flow through the column. During this procedure, IgG will bind to the column matrix. Other unbound serum components and protein will pass through the column and will be detected by the UV monitor. Continue to wash until all proteins have been eluted and the $A_{280}$ of the column eluate has returned to baseline. This usually takes 5 bed volumes of binding buffer but may take as many as 15 bed volumes.

### Sample Elution

7. Elution of bound antibody (IgG) should be accomplished with elution buffer at pH 3.0. Continuously monitor the $A_{280}$ of the eluate. Carefully wash the column with 5 bed volumes of buffer. Note the point at which elution buffer was added.

8. Since standing in low pH may damage antibodies, collect fractions in fraction collection tubes containing enough 1 M Tris HCl buffer (pH 9.0) to bring the pH back to a pH between 6 and 8. This may take as much as 2 ml of buffer.

## Regeneration of the Column

9. Regenerate the column after each use. If done properly, the column may be used for 10 to 12 separations with consistent results.
10. Wash the column with 5 bed volumes of regeneration buffer.
11. Finally, wash with 2 bed volumes of PBS containing 0.05% sodium azide. The bed material may be removed from the column and stored at 4° C until use later.

## Evaluation of Fractions

The student may now select various column fractions for determination of the presence of IgG. The same fractions should be saved for use in exercise 13. Use a modification of the ELISA procedure in the previous exercise.

12. Using a multichannel micropipette, fill rows B through H of a 96-well microtiter plate with 50 μl of coating buffer.
13. Carefully pipette 100 μl of the column fractions selected into wells A1 through A10. This will allow an assay of up to 10 fractions. Do not add antigen to well A11 and A12. These will serve as controls.
14. Serially dilute the sample by removing 50 μl from well A1 and placing it into well B1. Mix and remove 50 μl from B1 and place it into C1. Continue this procedure through well H1. Discard 50 μl from this well. Repeat this procedure for well A2 through A10 with other fractions using a new pipette tip.
15. Seal the plates with an adhesive cover and incubate overnight at 4° C.
16. After incubation, carefully remove the seal. Pour off the antigen solution by turning the plate over and shaking the liquid from the wells into the sink.
17. Fill each well with 200 μl of diluting buffer. Replace with a new piece of adhesive tape.
18. Incubate the microtiter plates at room temperature for 45 min.
19. At the end of the incubation period, remove the diluting buffer by pouring it into the sink.
20. Add 50 μl of diluted enzyme-labelled antibody conjugate to all wells of the plate. The appropriate dilution of conjugate should have been determined using the results from the previous ELISA exercise. Generally this dilution is between 1:200 and 1:800. The dilutions selected should show low background in controls and strong positive results with antigen.
21. Replace the adhesive cover and incubate for 45 min at 37° C.
22. At the end of the incubation period, remove the cover and pour and then shake the reagents into the sink.
23. Carefully wash the plate four times using wash buffer. Shake to remove the excess. Following the last wash, invert the plate over a paper towel and pat the plate dry.
24. Add 50 μl of the peroxidase substrate-buffer solution (*o*-phenylenediamine dihydrochloride) to each well and incubate at room temperature in the dark for 15 to 30 min. Check the plate for color every 5 min after the first 10 min of incubation. Stop color development by the addition of 1N HCl (as described in step 25) when color appears in wells containing antigen but the control wells remain colorless.
25. At the end of the incubation period, add 200 μl of 1N HCl to each well to stop the enzyme reaction.
26. Quickly pipette the mixture from each well of the microtiter plate into a 13 × 100 mm tube, add 3 ml of distilled water, and mix. Transfer this to a spectrophotometer tube.
27. Read the intensity of the color reaction in each tube in a spectrometer at $A_{495}$. Record the results. Use a microtiter plate reader for this step if one is available.

## Results

Record the spectrophotometric data collected during the elution procedure on a chart recorder or plot it on graph paper. Be sure to note the time when buffers were changed. If a flow-through monitor and automatic recording device were used, make appropriate corrections for the volume of liquid contained in the tubing between the monitor and fraction collector. Test the pH of fractions to make certain that it is between 6 and 8. If necessary, correct with 1M Tris HCl, pH 9.

Use the results to determine which fractions contain IgG and the relative amount of IgG in each fraction. Compare the results obtained from this part of the exercise with the graph generated on the chart recorder. Do you note any differences? If differences appear, how could they be explained?

## DISCUSSION

The profile obtained from continual UV monitoring of column effluent should indicate the point of separation of unbound protein from antibody. If the eluted antibody is to be stored for a prolonged period of time, it is essential that the pH of individual fractions be adjusted to neutrality. Adjustment will prevent the deterioration of the antibody and a subsequent inability of the antibody to perform in later assay procedures.

Comparison of the results produced by the UV monitor and ELISA may identify some differences. Graph both on the same paper and see when differences occur. How could differences in how these two methods "visualize" the IgG explain the point at which material is detected?

## SELECTED REFERENCES

Andrew, S. M., and J. A. Titus. 1991. Purification and fragmentation of antibodies. In *Current Protocols in Immunology.* Edited by J. E. Coligan, A. M. Kruisbeek, D. H. Margulies, E. M. Shevach, and W. Strober. p. 2.7.1–2.7.12. New York, NY: Greene Publishing and Wiley-Interscience.

*Bio-Rad Affi-Gel Protein A MAPS® II Instruction Manual.* Hercules, CA: Bio-Rad Laboratories.

Ey, P. L., S. J. Prowse, and C. R. Jenkin. 1978. Isolation of pure IgG1, IgG2a, and IgG2b immunoglobulins from mouse serum using protein A-Sepharose. *Immunochemistry.* 15:429.

Hardy, R. R. 1986. Purification and characterization of monoclonal antibodies. In *Handbook of Experimental Immunology.* Vol. 1: *Immunochemistry.* Edited by D. M. Weir. p 13.1–13.13. Oxford: Blackwell Scientific.

# SDS-Polyacrylamide Gel Electrophoresis (SDS-PAGE)

## INTRODUCTION

A variety of electrophoretic techniques can separate proteins in a mixture from one another for further analysis. One standard method is **polyacrylamide gel electrophoresis (PAGE)** under denaturing conditions. Another is accomplished in nondenaturing gels, and yet another uses gradient gels to separate proteins with a wide range of molecular weights. Regardless of the method selected, once separated, the resulting information helps determine the molecular size as well as the purity of individual proteins.

**One-dimensional electrophoresis** in a polyacrylamide gel provides an excellent way to accomplish separation of protein. The specific method chosen for this exercise, a de-

naturing discontinuous gel electrophoresis procedure, uses sodium dodecyl sulfate (SDS), a negatively charged detergent (Laemmli gel method).

The appropriate buffers have different pH values and generate a discontinuous pH as well as voltage gradient across the gel. The gradient thus formed tends to concentrate proteins into narrow bands, and they move through the gel. Since the gel contains 0.1% SDS, proteins tend to bind the SDS, thus neutralizing charge differences. Additionally, SDS causes unfolding of polypeptide chains, making these molecules freely soluble and readily electrophoresed (figure 13.1). The student may add 2-mercaptoethanol (2-ME) to reduce disulfide bonds and further solubilize

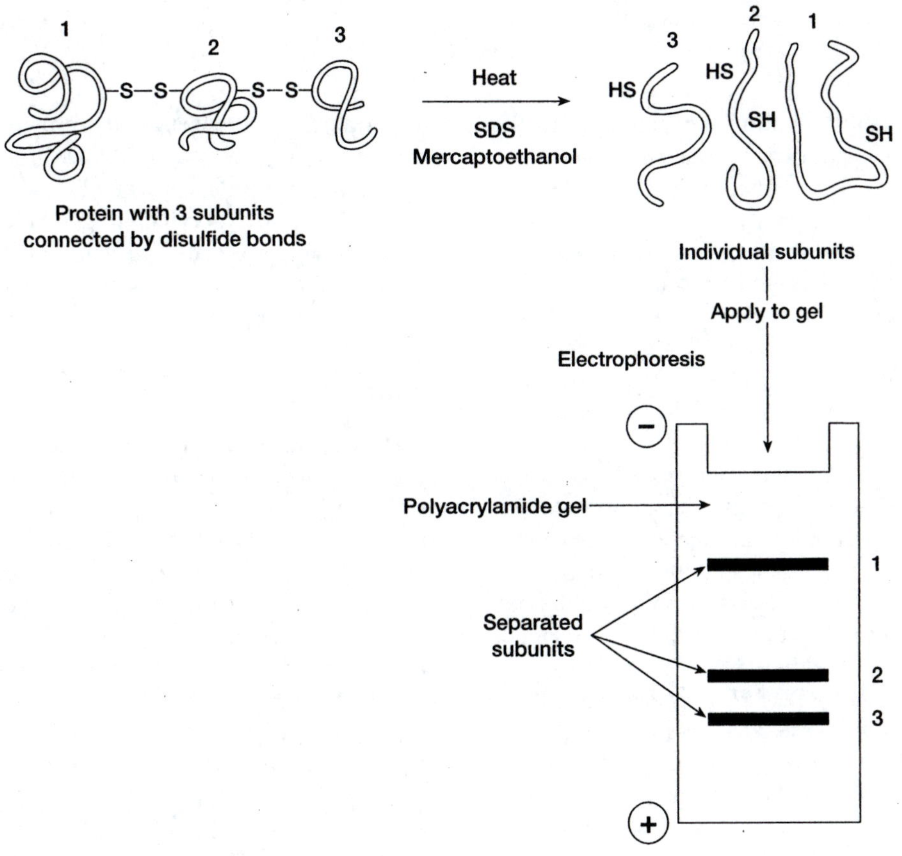

**FIGURE 13.1**
The procedure and results of SDS-PAGE.

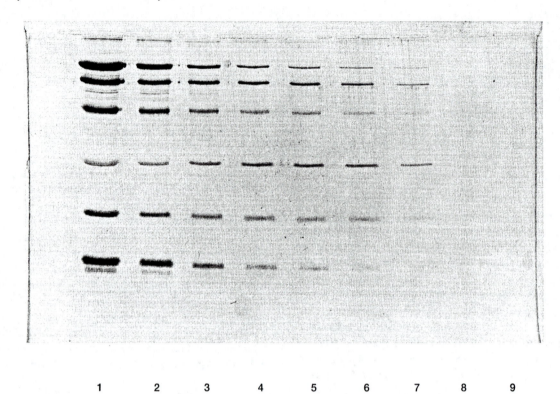

**FIGURE 13.2**
SDS-PAGE molecular weight standards run on a 7.5% gel and stained with Coomassie Blue R-250. Lanes from left to right contain serially diluted sample.
Courtesy Bio-Rad Laboratories, Life Science Group, Hercules, CA.

individual polypeptides. Migration proceeds toward the positive electrode when appropriate voltage is applied.

Separated proteins line up according to molecular weight and can be stained to make them visible. A commonly used stain is Coomassie Blue, but a silver stain can be used for increased sensitivity. Silver stain will detect as little as 10 ng of protein in a single band. **Prestained molecular weight standards** are normally run concurrently for comparative purposes. Figure 13.2 shows a photograph of the result of running molecular weight standards at various dilutions.

Basically, discontinuous polyacrylamide gels consist of a resolving (or lower) **separating gel** and an upper **stacking gel.** The stacking gel tends to concentrate large sample volumes, resulting in excellent resolution. Protein molecules in the sample then separate in the resolving gel. Polyacrylamide gels are made by polymerization of acrylamide and bis-acrylamide (N',N'methylene-bis-acrylamide). Polymerization is started by TEMED (tetramethylethylenediamine) and ammonium persulfate, which are considered to be initiators of the polymerization reaction. Polymerization results in a porous crosslinked polymer, and the porosity of the gel varies when the concentrations of specific reagents change.

In the following procedure, students utilize a Bio-Rad Mini Protean® II electrophoresis cell or a similar elec-trophoretic unit to separate the protein components (immunoglobulins) previously isolated from rabbit serum. To accomplish this, students will: (1) assemble electrophoretic units, (2) cast polyacrylamide gels, (3) load protein samples, (4) run the gel and (5) stain to determine separation. Proteins of known molecular weight will be run simultaneously for comparative purposes.

## SAFETY

Since electrophoresis involves the use of high voltage, DC electrical currents, students should remember that a **potential danger** exists. Always begin this exercise with the power supply turned off. Place the gels into the electrophoretic unit and close the unit according to the manufacturer's instructions. Insert the leads, and, following manufacturer's directions, increase the voltage or current to the desired level. Once the run finishes, turn off the power supply. Disconnect the leads and remove the gels.

Additionally, handle acrylamide with caution because repeated skin contact or inhalation may cause nervous system disorders. Always wear gloves and work in a ventilated hood when working with acrylamide. Do not pipette by mouth. Be sure to wash hands and skin that have come in direct contact with acrylamide with soap and rinse thoroughly with water.

## MATERIALS

Prepare the following using formulations given in the appendix prior to beginning the exercise: running (electrode) buffer, pH 8.3 (5X stock), sample buffer (SDS reducing buffer), Coomassie Blue stain, destain solution, gel-preserving solution, 1.5 M Tris-HCl, pH 8.8, 0.5 M Tris-HCl, pH 6.8 and 10% SDS. Procedures for *stacking gel* and *separating gel* preparation appear in the appropriate step in the procedure.

  Bio-Rad Mini Protean® II electrophoresis system

  Eluted fractions (samples) from the Protein A chromatography procedure in exercise 12

  Glass slides (large and small)

  0.75-mm spacers

  Leveling bubble

  Gel casting stand

  Power supply

  Power cords

  Separating gel

  Vacuum pump

  50-ml Erlenmeyer side arm flasks

Teflon comb

TEMED

10% Ammonium persulfate (prepare immediately before use)

18-gauge needles and 5-ml syringes

Micropipette and tips

Small test tubes

Cellophane

Prestained molecular weight standards

## PROCEDURE

1. The following procedure describes the use of the Mini-Protean® II cell. Figure 13.3, a photograph of this system, shows the major components. However, a number of electrophoretic cells provide excellent results, but procedures for equipment setup may vary. Students should carefully follow instructions for assembly of the cell. When assembled, the cell can run two slab gels for analysis of as many as thirty samples and the electrophoretic run can be completed within 45 min.

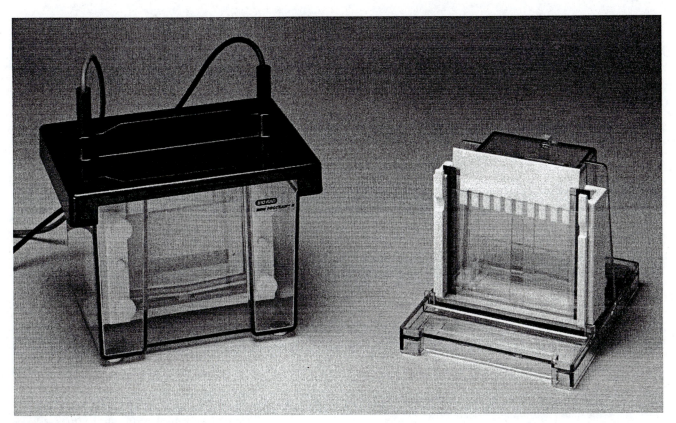

**FIGURE 13.3**
The Mini-Protean® II cell. The buffer chamber and lid are shown on the left with the inner cooling core inserted. The sandwich clamp assembly positioned on the casting stand appears on the right.
Courtesy Bio-Rad Laboratories, Life Science Group, Hercules, CA.

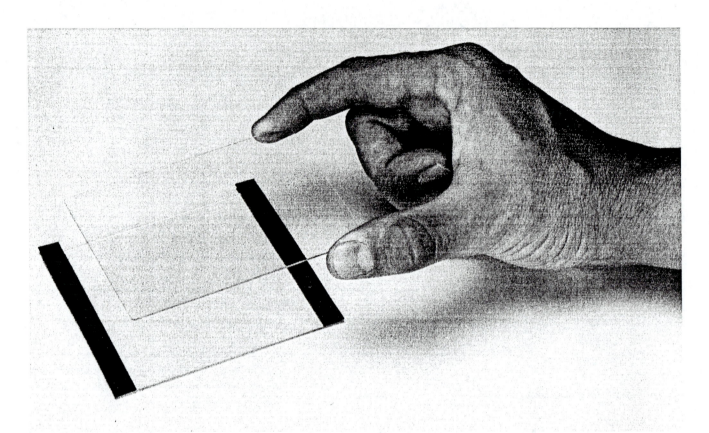

**FIGURE 13.4**
Beginning the assembly of the gel sandwich.
Courtesy Bio-Rad Laboratories, Life Science Group, Hercules, CA.

## Assembling Glass Plate Sandwiches

2. Lay the larger rectangular glass plate down on a clean, dry surface. Place two spacers of equal thickness along the short edges.
3. Next, place the shorter glass plate on top of the spacers. Align the bottom ends of the spacers with the bottom of the glass plates. The spacers will protrude above the top of the larger plate (figure 13.4).
4. Make sure that the four screws on the clamp assembly are loose. Stand the clamp assembly up so that the screws face away from you, and place the clamp assembly into the casting stand.
5. Firmly grasp the glass plate sandwich with the larger plate away from you and carefully slide it into the clamp assembly. The larger glass plate should be against the acrylic pressure plate of the clamp assembly (figure 13.5).
6. If the spacers are not flush against the sides of the clamp assembly, relocate them properly.

Tighten the screws of the clamp assembly until the plates and spacers are held securely in position.
7. Using a leveling bubble, level the casting stand with the alignment slot facing you. Make sure the removable gray silicone gaskets are clean and properly aligned. (If the gaskets are dirty or misaligned, a bad seal will result and the assembly may leak.)
8. Transfer the clamp assembly to one of the casting slots in the casting stand. If two gels are to be cast, place the clamp assembly on the side opposite the alignment slot. This allows for an easier adjustment of the next plate assembly.
9. Attach the plate assembly by placing the acrylic plate against the wall of the casting slot at the bottom so that the glass plates rest on the rubber gasket. Snap the acrylic plate under the overhang of the casting slot by pressing on the white portion of the clamps. Do not push against the glass plates themselves (figure 13.6).

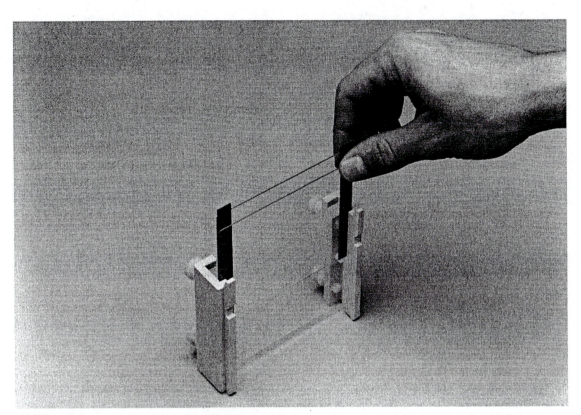

**FIGURE 13.5**
Insertion of the glass plate sandwich into the clamp assembly.
Courtesy Bio-Rad Laboratories, Life Science Group, Hercules, CA.

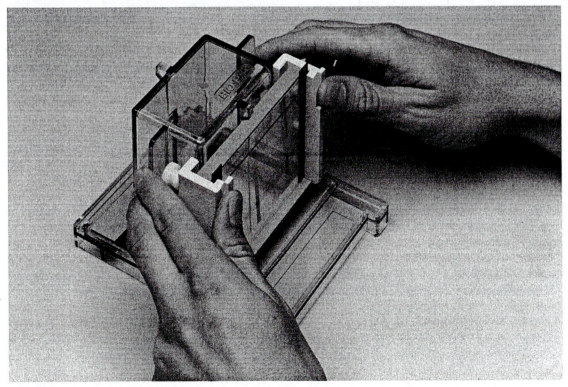

**FIGURE 13.6**
Attachment of plate assembly to the casting stand.
Courtesy Bio-Rad Laboratories, Life Science Group, Hercules, CA.

*Casting the Gels*

10. Prepare components for the *separating gel* according to the following directions (12% monomer in 0.375M Tris, pH 8.8): Prepare the acrylamide/bis (30% stock) by weighing out 30.0 g of acrylamide and 0.8 g N'-N'-bis-methylene-acrylamide. Place these in a flask and add distilled water to 100 ml. Filter and store in the dark at 4° C. Alternatively, premixed acrylamide/bis may be purchased from a variety of suppliers.

11. Dissolve 10 g SDS in 100 ml of water and set it aside.

12. Using the following formulation, prepare the *separating gel* in a 50 ml Erlenmeyer side arm flask. This will provide enough material for one minigel.
    a. 3.5 ml distilled water
    b. 2.5 ml 1.5M Tris-HCl (pH 8.8)
    c. 100 μl 10% (w/v) SDS
    d. 4.0 ml acrylamide/bis (30% stock)

13. Place a rubber stopper on the flask and degas with a vacuum pump for 15 min at room temperature.

14. While degassing the separating gel, weigh out 0.1 g ammonium persulfate in a clean, dry test tube. This will be added to the separating gel only when degassing is complete. Why?

15. Put the well-forming comb into the assembled gel sandwich. Place a mark on the glass plate 1 cm below the teeth of the comb. This important step marks the level to which separating gel is poured.

16. After degassing, add 5 μl of TEMED into the separating gel and swirl gently.

17. Add 1.0 ml distilled water to the ammonium persulfate, mix, and add 50 μl of this to the flask. Gently swirl the entire mixture until complete mixing is accomplished. From this point on, students should work quickly so that the monomer does not polymerize in the flask.

18. Complete the preparation of the gel sandwich by pouring the gel. Draw up the gel into a 5 ml syringe with an 18-gauge needle and apply at one edge of the larger plate between the gel sandwich. Add the gel smoothly to prevent mixing with air and add up to the mark made previously.

19. Immediately after the gel has been poured, overlay with distilled water. Do this with a needle and syringe and deliver the water with a steady rate to prevent mixing with the gel. This step provides an even edge to the separating gel and prevents air from coming in contact with the gel.

20. The polymerization of the gel should take 45 min to 1 hr. Periodically check the monomer left in the side arm flask to determine the time of polymerization.

*Stacking Gel Preparation*

21. The *stacking gel* can be prepared during the final stages of separating gel polymerization. Prepare components for the stacking gel according to the following directions (4% gel, 0.12M Tris, pH 6.8). Add the following to a 50 ml Erlenmeyer side arm flask. This provides enough material for one minigel.
    a. 6.1 ml distilled water
    b. 2.5 ml 0.5M Tris-HCl, pH 6.8
    c. 100 μl 10% (w/v) SDS
    d. 1.3 ml acrylamide/bis (30% stock)

22. Place a rubber stopper on the flask and degas with a vacuum pump for 15 min at room temperature.

23. While degassing, make a fresh 10% solution of ammonium persulfate as described in step 14.

24. During the last few minutes of degassing, remove the water layered over the separating gel. Simply tip the plate assembly upside down over a paper towel.

25. When the degassing procedure is complete, add 10 μl of TEMED and 50 μl of the 10% ammonium persulfate solution. Swirl gently to mix.

26. Using a 5-ml syringe and an 18-gauge needle, add the stacking gel to the sandwich. Place it between the glass plates to fill the space between the separating gel and the top of the short glass plate.

27. **Important:** Immediately after pouring the gel, insert the comb between the plates. Insert at a 20° angle to help prevent air bubbles from being trapped beneath the comb teeth.

28. Allow the stacking gel to polymerize for 30 min. The gel may shrink as polymerization occurs. Add distilled water to the stacking gel if this happens.

29. After polymerization is complete, carefully remove the comb. Fill the wells that have been formed with distilled water.

30. Remove the water and overlay the gel with **running buffer.** Immediately remove the running buffer and add a fresh overlay of the same buffer. The resulting completed gel should resemble figure 13.7.

31. Lay the inner cooling core down and carefully slide the clamp-assembly wedges underneath the slots on the inner cooling core. The inner glass plate of the gel sandwich should butt against the notch of the U-shaped gasket. Snap the clamp assembly unto the cooling core until the latch engages (figure 13.8).

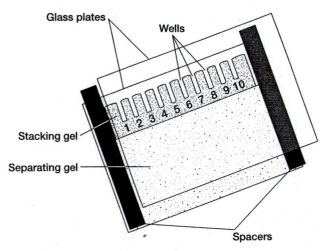

**FIGURE 13.7**
A complete gel sandwich ready for sample application.

### Preparing Samples

32. Transfer 10 µl of the sample selected from those eluted from the affinity chromatography column in exercise 12 into a small test tube. Add 30 µl of sample buffer to each tube.
33. Transfer 100 µl of prestained standards to a separate tube but do not add sample buffer to the standards.
34. Incubate all tubes at 95° C for 5 min. Why? Following incubation they are ready to load onto the stacking gel.

### Loading the Samples

35. Load the samples *under* the running buffer. This may be accomplished with an Eppendorf-type pipetter and a thin gel-loading tip, a needle and syringe, or a Hamilton syringe. If non-disposable equipment is used, make sure to carefully clean between each sample. Carefully, transfer 5 µl of each sample to a different well. Use wells numbered 1, 3 through 8, and 10. Layer the sample between the glass plates within 2 to 3 mm of the bottom of the well. Slowly dispense the sample (figure 13.9).

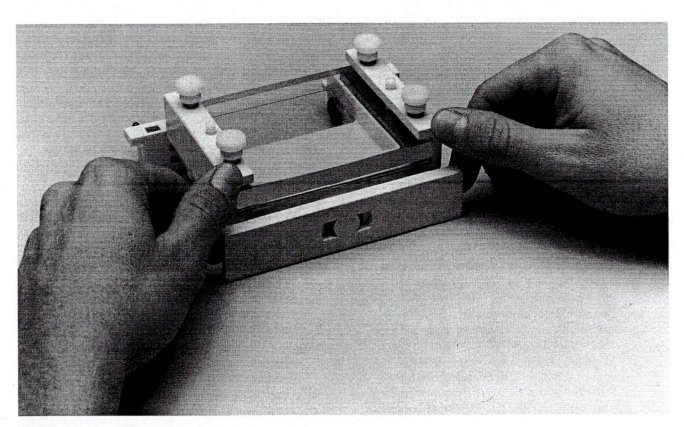

**FIGURE 13.8**
Insertion of the clamp assembly with gel sandwich into the inner cooling core.
Courtesy Bio-Rad Laboratories, Life Science Group, Hercules, CA.

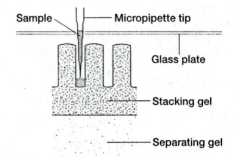

**FIGURE 13.9**
Application of the sample to a well in the stacking gel.

36. Place the prestained standard in wells 2 and 9. This facilitates a determination of molecular weight.

*Preparation of Buffer Chambers*

37. Lower the inner cooling core into the lower buffer chamber. Add 115 ml of **running (electrode) buffer** to the upper buffer chamber. **Important:** Fill with buffer until the buffer reaches a level halfway between the short and long plates. Do not overfill.

38. Pour electrode buffer into the lower buffer chamber so that the bottom 1 cm of the gel is covered.

*Running the Gel*

39. Place the lid on top of the lower buffer chamber. Make the proper connection by matching the colors of the plugs with the jacks on the electrophoretic unit.

40. Connect the electrophoresis unit to the power supply.

41. Run at 200V for 45 to 60 min. Stop electrophoresis when the bromphenol blue (tracking dye) is about 1 cm from the bottom of the gel. Remember that this tracking dye was added to the sample buffer.

42. Turn the power supply off, disconnect the power cords, and remove the chamber lid.

43. Lift out the plate assembly and clamp and remove the plate assembly from the clamp.

44. Disassemble the plate assembly. Remove the spacers and use one of them to scrape away the stacking gel. Discard the stacking gel.

45. Mark the upper right hand corner of the separating gel with a razor blade for reference. Place the separating gel into a container and cover with Coomassie Blue stain. Cover the container and store overnight at room temperature .

46. After overnight incubation, pour off the stain and replace with destain solution. The Coomassie Blue staining solution may be reused.

47. Rotate on a platform rotator until the gel clears. This may take several washes with destain solution.

48. To dry and preserve the gel, soak cellophane and the gel in gel-preserving solution for 5 min. Sandwich the gel between cellophane layers and place on a drying rack. Drying time may be as long as 2 days.

## Results

Measure the distance from the top of the separating gel to the middle of each standard. Plot this information on semi-log paper. This will produce a **standard curve.** Measure the distance migrated by each band in the sample lanes. Use the standard curve to determine the molecular weight of each protein found in the sample lanes.

## DISCUSSION

The combination of polyacrylamide gel electrophoresis and SDS results in a powerful tool for the determination of purity and molecular weight. This exercise produces the separation of individual molecules from a complex, crude mixture. In addition, the incorporation of standard proteins of known molecular weight allows the student to generate a standard curve. The molecular weight of individual unknown proteins may be interpolated from the standard curve. This **analytical tool** may also be used to observe the development of specific proteins within a biological system over time. In addition, the primary structure of proteins from different sources may be examined by limited enzymatic digestion of purified proteins and subsequent SDS-PAGE.

## SELECTED REFERENCES

*Bio-Rad Mini Protean® II Instruction Manual.* Hercules, CA: Bio-Rad Laboratories.

Gallagher, S. R., and J. A. Smith. 1991. Electrophoretic separation of proteins. In *Current Protocols in Immunology.* Edited by J. E. Coligan, A. M. Kruisbeek, D. H. Margulies, E. M. Shevach, and W. Strober. p. 8.4.1–8.4.21. New York, NY: Greene Publishing and Wiley-Interscience.

Hames, B. D., and D. Rickwood, eds. 1981. Gel electrophoresis of proteins. New York, NY: Oxford University Press.

Laemmli, U. K. 1970. Cleavage of structural proteins during the assembly of the head of bacteriophage T4. *Nature* (Lond.) 227:680.

# 14

# *Western Blotting*

## INTRODUCTION

In 1975, Southern first reported blotting as a procedure. DNA was transferred from agarose gels to nitrocellulose membranes, and, since then, RNA and protein have been blotted to a variety of binding membranes.

**Western blotting** (immunoblotting), a rapid and sensitive method, uses antibodies to detect the presence of small amounts of antigens in complex mixtures. The antibodies, either monoclonal or polyclonal, recognize specific epitopes on the homologous antigen. Often Western blotting is combined with **SDS-PAGE.** Protein molecules, first isolated on the basis of molecular weight with SDS-PAGE, are then electrophoretically transferred to a nitrocellulose membrane. On the nitrocellulose membrane a protein can be detected with specific antibody conjugated to horseradish peroxidase or other enzyme. The protein appears visible when the conjugate is incubated with the enzyme's substrate.

This technique can detect a specific protein in a complex mixture of molecules or a specific antibody in a serum sample. However, the procedure has limitations. The transfer of protein may be ineffective, or denatured protein may not be recognized by the antibody. Controls should be run concurrently to obtain consistent results that can be interpreted properly. In addition, it is important to select a substrate which produces an insoluble product after reaction with the enzyme. When performed properly, this powerful procedure results in a colored band which is obvious on the white nitrocellulose membrane.

The Western blot procedure as described is a **continuation of the SDS-PAGE** separation procedure in the previous exercise. The procedure utilizes the Bio-Rad Mini Trans-Blot® Electrophoretic Transfer Cell. The separated protein will be transferred to a protein-binding membrane. Two of the lanes in the gel should be molecular weight standards to allow the generation of a standard curve and to verify the transfer of prestained standards to the membrane.

## MATERIALS

Prepare the following using formulations given in the appendix prior to beginning the exercise: transfer buffer, pH 8.3, blocking buffer, pH 7.5, Tris buffered saline, wash buffer.

Bio-Rad Mini Trans-Blot® Electrophoretic Transfer Cell

Eluted fractions (samples) from the Protein A chromatography procedure or polyacrylamide gel from the SDS-PAGE exercise (exercise 13)

Some materials from previous exercises on affinity chromatography and SDS-PAGE

Nitrocellulose membrane

Filter paper

Filter pads

Latex gloves

Forceps

Scissors

Containers for staining

Anti-rabbit IgG peroxidase conjugate (1:100 dilution in blocking buffer)

Substrate (*o*-phenylenediamine dihydrochloride) for conjugated enzyme

Magnetic stirrer

## PROCEDURE

1. Follow the safety procedures outlined in exercise 13.
2. Prepare the Bio-Ice cooling unit by filling with distilled water and freezing prior to the transfer procedure. This prevents overheating in the electrophoretic cell during electrophoresis.
3. Prepare the buffers prior to beginning the procedure and store at 4° C. The temperature of the buffers should be 4° C at the start of the transfer.
4. Complete the SDS-PAGE procedure on samples eluted from the Protein A affinity column as described in exercise 13.
5. After electrophoresis, remove the gels from the plate assembly and separate from the stacking gel.
6. Rinse the gels in transfer buffer to remove all electrophoresis buffer salts and detergents and leave them in transfer buffer until ready to use. This step is important.

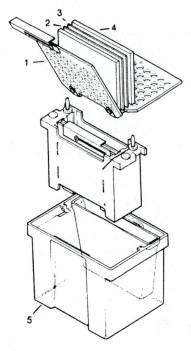

**FIGURE 14.1**
**Locking gel cassette clamping system.** The cassette (1) holds
the gel (2) and membrane (3) while fiber pads and filter paper (4) on
both sides provide positive contact within the gel sandwich. The gel
cassette is inserted vertically in the buffer tank (5).
Courtesy Bio-Rad Laboratories, Life Science Group, Hercules, CA.

7. Wear gloves and cut the nitrocellulose
membrane to the dimensions of the gel and label
the orientation of the gel. Use forceps to handle
the membrane when appropriate.

8. Soak a precut nitrocellulose membrane in a
separate container of transfer buffer. This may
take up to 30 min for complete wetting. Also
soak precut filter paper (two per gel) and fiber
pads in transfer buffer. **Note:** Avoid trapping air
bubbles in the filter paper or pads because air
bubbles can block the transfer of molecules.

9. Place the Mini Trans-Blot® electrode in the buffer
chamber. Fill the buffer tank half full with transfer
buffer. Place a magnetic stirbar in the bottom of
the unit. (Important: Rinse the buffer chamber
thoroughly with distilled water before use.)

*Cassette Assembly*

10. The cassette assembly holds the gel, the
membrane, fiber pads and filter paper
(figure 14.1).

11. Place the cassette into a shallow dish with the
grey-colored panel (cathode side) down and the
clear panel (anode side) resting against the wall
of the vessel.

12. Place a presoaked fiber pad on the gray panel.
Center the pad as well as all components that
follow.

13. Place a piece of saturated filter paper on top of
the fiber pad. Pipette approximately 3 ml of
transfer buffer onto the filter paper.

14. Place the polyacrylamide gel with separated
protein on top of the paper. Again, center all
components so that nothing extends past the
edge of the cassette. Be sure that no air bubbles
are trapped between the gel and filter paper.

15. Pipette 5 ml of transfer buffer onto the gel and
place the presoaked nitrocellulose membrane
onto the gel. Roll a glass rod (pipette) over the
membrane to exclude air bubbles that may have
formed.

16. Pipette 5 ml of transfer buffer onto the
nitrocellulose membrane and then complete the
sandwich by placing a presoaked filter paper
onto the membrane and then a presoaked fiber
pad onto the filter paper.

17. Close the cassette. Two cassettes may be
prepared for a single run.

18. Place the gel holders into the buffer tank. The
grey electrode must face the black cathode panel
of the Mini Trans-Blot® cell.

19. Place the frozen Bio-Ice cooling block into the
buffer chamber.

20. Add cold transfer buffer to just above the top
row of circles on the gel-holder cassette.

21. Place the buffer tank on a magnetic stirrer.
Connect the lead to the buffer chamber and insert
the leads into the power supply.

22. Increase the voltage to 100 V and run for 1 hr.
Review safety procedures given in exercise 13.

*Staining and Blotting of the Nitrocellulose Membrane*

23. At the end of the electrophoresis run, turn off the
power and unplug the power supply. Remove the
gels and the nitrocellulose membrane from the
gel-holder cassette.

24. Carefully, peel the nitrocellulose membrane from
the gel and mark the membrane in relation to the
gel for future reference. If you used prestained
standards, transfer of these to the nitrocellulose
during the process just completed indicates a
successful procedure. Congratulations if you can
see the prestained standards on the nitrocellulose
membrane—you have performed a successful
transfer! Discard the gels.

25. Place one of the nitrocellulose membranes into a
container with 40 ml of blocking buffer for 30
min at room temperature. The membrane may be

stored in blocking buffer at 4° C for up to 1 week. What is the purpose of this step?

26. Remove the blocking buffer from the container and add 20 ml of blocking buffer containing 200 µl diluted antibody (anti-rabbit IgG peroxidase conjugate, 1:100 dilution). Incubate for 1 to 2 hr at room temperature or overnight at 4° C.

27. After incubation, wash the nitrocellulose membrane 5 times with wash buffer using the following procedure:
   a. Complete one 5 min wash with 150 ml of wash buffer. Use a platform shaker.
   b. Wash 4 additional times with 150 ml of wash buffer. Start with a 5 min wash and increase the time with every wash so that the last wash is 10 min long.

28. Add approximately 50 ml of the substrate solution (see the ELISA exercise in exercise 11 for the procedure for substrate preparation) to the washed nitrocellulose membrane. The membrane should remain in the substrate solution until color development appears.

29. Finally, wash the membrane with distilled water and place on a paper towel to dry.

## Results

Measure the distance (in millimeters) migrated by the prestained standards starting at the top of the gel. Use the values obtained and the molecular weights of these to construct a **standard curve.** The instructor will give you information about the MW of the standards. The values should be plotted on semilog paper as log molecular weight versus distance migrated. The molecular weights of molecules stained with conjugated antibodies may then be determined by using the standard curve. Explain. Figure 14.2 provides an example of molecular weight standards transferred to nitrocellulose. The molecular weights vary from 97,000 for phosphorylase b (at the top of the first 2 lanes) to 14,400 for lysozyme at the bottom. The protein was stained with colloidal gold total protein stain.

## DISCUSSION

The Western blot procedure, coupled with specific immunostaining, provides a powerful tool for the identification of specific epitopes. Both clinical and research laboratories use the procedure to determine the presence, relative motility, and concentration of individual proteins and protein fragments. In addition, it can determine if antibodies with specific reactivity are present in a serum sample or if the patient has been exposed to a specific immunogen.

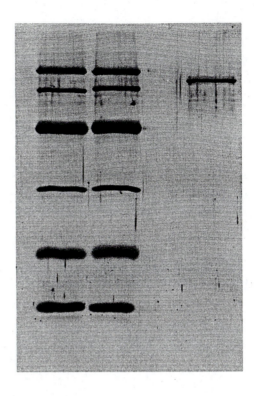

**1        2        3        4**

**FIGURE 14.2**
The result of a sample in a 12% SDS-polyacrylamide gel that was electrophoresed and transferred to nitrocellulose. Lane 1 shows biotinylated SDS-PAGE standards; lane 2 contains SDS-PAGE molecular weight standards; lane 3 is blank; lane 4 contains human transferrin.
Courtesy Bio-Rad Laboratories, Life Science Group, Hercules, CA.

## SELECTED REFERENCES

Blake, M. S., H. Johnston, G. V. Rullel Jones, and E. C. Gotschlich. 1974. A rapid, sensitive method for detection of alkaline phosphatase-conjugated antiantibody on Western blots. *Anal. Biochem.* 136:175.

Burnette, W. H. 1981. Western blotting: Electrophoretic transfer of proteins from SDS-poly-acrylamide gels to unmodified nitrocellulose and radiographic detection with antibody and radioiodinated protein A. *Anal. Biochem.* 112:195.

Harlow, E., and D. Lane. 1988. Immunoblotting. In *Antibodies: A laboratory manual.* p. 473. Cold Spring Harbor, NY: Cold Spring Harbor Laboratory.

McCafferty, J., A. D. Griffiths, G. Winter, and D. J. Chiswell. 1990. Phage antibodies: Filamentous phage displaying antibody variable domains. *Nature.* 348:552.

Winston, S. E., S. A. Fuller, and J. G. R. Hurrell. 1991. In *Current protocols in immunology.* Edited by J. E. Coligan, A. M. Kruisbeek, D. H. Margulies, E. M. Shevach, and W. Strober. p. 8.10.1–8.10.5. New York, NY: Greene Publishing and Wiley-Interscience.

# *Cell Techniques*

Section IV concentrates on the **culture of immune cells** and the measurement of their activities in culture. The cell culturist desires to maintain cells in vitro by providing conditions in the laboratory that replicate as closely as possible those present in the living animal. These conditions include a solid surface, the appropriate nutrients, and the proper pH and temperature. If requirements are met, some cells will reproduce and perhaps differentiate. Immune cells, like most other vertebrate cells, stop growth and die after a specific number of cell divisions in culture. However, with appropriate methods the student can collect sufficient data to make conclusions about the function of immune cells before the cells die. The exercises in section IV teach these methods.

The first exercise describes a procedure for culturing **murine spleen cells.** This exercise makes use of a mitogen, a substance that provokes cells to divide. Lipopolysaccharide, a B cell mitogen, will be added to stimulate cell division and, at specific times, viability and proliferation of the spleen cell population will be determined. This important exercise provides cell culture fundamentals necessary for the experiments that follow.

Once the student can handle cell culture, exercises that follow utilize cell culture methods to derive specific information about cells. Two exercises prompt students to work with various populations of lymphocytes for the purpose of identifying **subpopulations** of lymphocytes. In the first, a fluorescent antibody detects surface immunoglobulin on **B cells,** a method that allows these cells to be distinguished from other lymphocytes in a spleen cell population. **T cells** in peripheral blood are distinguished with a rosette technique.

**Mitogens** are important and useful tools for the immunologist; exercise 18 provides a method for detecting the effect of a specific mitogen on spleen cells. Spleen cells in culture will be treated with Concanvalin A and fed a radiolabeled DNA precursor. Proliferation of spleen cells that was initiated by the mitogen is determined after an incubation period. The determination is made by observing the incorporation of the radiolabeled precursor into DNA of the daughter cells.

The final exercise in this section shows that immune cells can **communicate** via soluble molecules. It uses a culture vessel to separate immune cell populations by only a semipermeable membrane, making it impossible for them to come in direct contact with each other. If one cell type is influenced by soluble mediators produced by the other, the influence (e.g., stimulation of blastogenesis) can be detected by measurement of cell proliferation.

*Figure IV presents the approximate instructor preparation time and student laboratory time necessary for successful completion of exercises 15 through 19.*

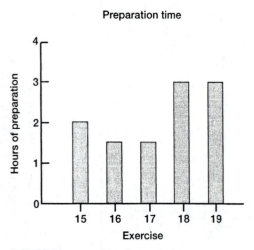

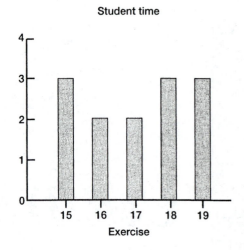

**FIGURE IV**
Time allocation for Section IV exercises.

# 15

# *Cell Culture*

## INTRODUCTION

The fact that a single cell comprises only one small part of a larger organism makes its activities difficult to study. For this reason, more than 75 years ago researchers considered the possibility of culturing **single cells** in vitro, but not until the 1950s did cell culture techniques become sufficiently sophisticated that cultured cells could be maintained and utilized routinely.

Some cells can replicate only a few times free of the animal body, but others seem to replicate indefinitely. Cultures of cells taken directly from animals, called **primary cultures,** are capable of limited growth. Primary cultures in some cases can be subcultured and are then called **secondary cultures. Diploid cell strains** may replicate as many as 100 times before they die, but **continuous cell lines** can propagate indefinitely. Continuous cell lines may be referred to as **established cell lines.**

All cultured cells require a solid matrix such as glass or plastic for growth and differentiation to occur, and when cultured properly, display many of the differentiated properties of the tissue from which they were derived. Lympho-cytes, phagocytes, and ancillary cells have been cultured in vitro, and the contributions of each or combinations of them to the overall immune response have been clarified.

Chemically defined media greatly aid the in vitro culture of cells. A cell culture medium has all the nutrients required by cells, including amino acids, vitamins, salts, and other growth factors such as glucose, and, in most media, whole serum. Other substances like antibiotics and pH indicators may also be added. Most media are buffered to pH 7.4.

The medium chosen for use in this exercise is RPMI 1640. Originally designed for the culture of human leukocytes, it can be used routinely to culture spleen cells. It contains inorganic salts, amino acids, vitamins, glucose, reduced glutathione, and phenol red. It may be prepared in the laboratory but is usually purchased from a vendor in the liquid or powdered form. For this exercise, 5% fetal calf serum will be added to provide additional growth factors to assure the continued viability of the cultured cells. Additional substances may also be added; for example, the addition of 2-mercaptoethanol enhances in vitro responses of spleen cells and allows the cells to be cultured at lower cell density. The exact reason is unknown.

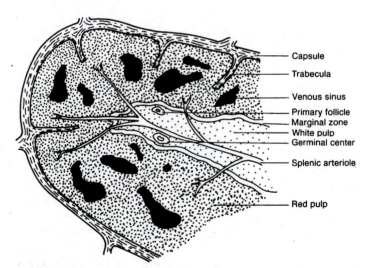

**FIGURE 15.1**
A diagrammatic representation of the functional areas of the spleen. Blood enters through the splenic arterioles which are surrounded by a lymphoid sheath that comprises the thymus dependent area. Follicles are dispersed throughout and represent the B dependent areas that become germinal centers to provide the humoral response when stimulated. The red pulp contains erythrocytes, macrophages and the venous sinusoids.

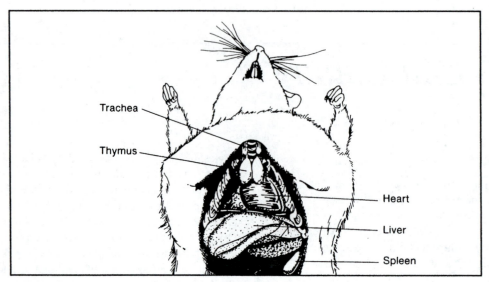

**FIGURE 15.2**
The location of the thymus and spleen in a young mouse.

The immune cells of the spleen serve as useful tools for the immunologist. They are found principally in the white pulp which usually surrounds the arterial vessels of the spleen (figure 15.1). In this exercise, lipopolysaccharide (LPS), a B cell mitogen, will be added as a stimulus to induce some of these cells to differentiate.

This exercise provides the student with the methodology necessary to explant and culture immune tissue. Cells from the spleen will be cultured and **viability and proliferation** determined. These procedures, when mastered, will be useful in exercises that follow.

## MATERIALS

(Per pair)

    1 mouse

    $CO_2$ for mouse euthanasia

    Surgical instruments (forceps, scissors, scalpel)

    70% ethyl alcohol

    95% ethyl alcohol

    Plastic Petri dish (sterile, 100 × 15 mm)

    RPMI 1640 medium prepared according to
        manufacturer's instructions. Add 200 micromolar
        2-mercaptoethanol, 35 µg LPS/ml, 7 µg/ml
        dextran sulfate, 5% fetal calf serum and 100 U/ml
        penicillin and 100 µg/ml streptomycin

    Rubber policeman (sterile)

    Sterile capillary pipettes

    Sterile centrifuge tubes

    Unopette® white cell pipette and diluting fluid

    Hemacytometer

    Sterile tubes for dilution series

    Culture tubes (sterile)

    35 × 10-mm culture dishes

    Ice bath

    Trypan Blue stain solution

    Phosphate buffered saline (PBS)

    1-ml pipettes

    5-ml pipettes

    Biological safety cabinet

    $CO_2$ incubator (37° C)

    Vortex mixer

    Filter for sterilization of media

## PROCEDURE

1. Obtain 8- to 12-week-old mice and kill them according to instructions given in exercise 4 for mouse euthanasia. Each pair of students should use one mouse.

2. Use a biological safety cabinet (laminar flow hood) if one is available for the procedures that follow to lessen the chance for microbial contamination. Since spleen cells will be cultured for an extended period of time, contamination would be detrimental to the cultured cells.

3. Use sterile surgical instruments and aseptic techniques for the splenectomy. Aseptic technique includes wetting the abdominal area with 70% ethyl alcohol prior to making the incision. Make the incision in the inguinal region and reflect the skin to expose the peritoneal wall.

Make another incision in the peritoneum directly above the spleen. The spleen is easily identified as a long, flat, dark red organ. Pull it through the abdominal incision with sterile forceps and cut it away from the connecting tissues. See figure 15.2 for the location of the spleen.

4. Put the spleen in a sterile Petri dish containing 5 ml of prewarmed medium. The medium used in this and some exercises to follow is RPMI 1640. For this exercise it should contain 200 micromolar 2-mercaptoethanol, 35 $\mu$g/ml bacterial lipopolysaccharide (LPS) and 7 $\mu$g/ml dextran sulfate, plus 5% fetal calf serum. Add 100 U/ml penicillin and 100 $\mu$g/ml streptomycin to retard bacterial growth.

5. Make a longitudinal cut in the spleen with a sterile scalpel or razor blade and tease out the cells with a sterile rubber policeman. This should produce a suspension of single cells. Do these procedures carefully but quickly. Drying means sure loss of viability.

6. Tilt the dish and remove **suspended cells** (not clumps of cells or connective tissue) with a sterile capillary pipette and put into a sterile centrifuge tube. Centrifuge at $250 \times g$ for 5 min.

7. Discard the supernatant and add an additional 5 ml of medium. Resuspend the cells gently with a vortex mixer. Centrifuge again at $250 \times g$ for 5 min. Discard the supernatant.

8. Finally, resuspend the cells in 1 ml of cold medium and hold the cells in an ice bath until needed. Carefully note dilution factors from this point on so that an accurate cell count is possible.

9. Determine the cell count by preparing a 1:20 dilution using a Unopette® white cell pipette and diluting fluid as described in exercise 3. Add to a hemacytometer, count, and determine the number of cells/ml of the spleen cell suspension.

10. Dilute to $3 \times 10^5$ cells/ml in RPMI 1640. Prepare at least 12 ml to provide enough of the cell suspension for four cell cultures as well as material for viability determinations. An explanation of cell dilution appears in the appendix.

11. Dispense 2.5 ml of the diluted cell suspension into each of 4, $35 \times 10$-mm plastic culture dishes. Incubate all cell suspensions at $37°$ C in a 5% $CO_2$ humid atmosphere. Return the excess cell suspension to the ice bath.

12. Test the remaining suspension from step 11 for viability. Use the **Trypan Blue exclusion** method described in the next step. Find the methods for preparation of Trypan Blue solution and phosphate buffered saline in the appendix.

13. Pipette exactly 0.2 ml of the cell suspension from step 11 into a culture tube. Add an equal volume of the Trypan Blue stain (prepared on the day to be used) and mix gently. This makes a 1:2 dilution of cells. Add these stained cells to a hemacytometer and count the **total number** of cells and also the number of **nonviable** cells. Nonviable cells are blue because these cells cannot keep stain from diffusing into the cell, while viable cells exclude the stain. The total number should agree with the value obtained in step 10.

14. Count cells daily throughout the duration of the experiment in order to maintain the **proper number** of cells in the cultures.

15. To do this, the cultured spleen cells must be **subcultured** (split) at regular intervals. Count the cells on a daily basis, and every time the cell density reaches 1.5 to $2 \times 10^6$ cells/ml, dilute 2.5 ml of cell suspension 1:2 in fresh culture medium and plate in a new sterile $35 \times 10$-mm Petri dish.

16. Determine the increase in number of cells for a period of 7 days. Also determine the viability of the cells by the Trypan Blue method each time a cell count is performed.

17. Plot the **increase in cell number** over the 7-day incubation period. The plotted values (total number of cells) approximate the numbers of cells that would have been found in the culture plates had the cultures been diluted and not split. Relate cell viability to the increase in cell numbers.

## DISCUSSION

LPS serves as a B cell mitogen to encourage replication of lymphocytes. Researchers frequently use LPS to trigger B cell differentiation. About 35 percent of all B cells can be activated by LPS to produce IgM, but less than 4 percent will be activated to produce IgG. Dextran sulfate also acts as a mitogen in this exercise.

Strictly follow the outlined procedures for best results. The methods presented will assist the student for future cell culture and apply to all cultured cells, not just lymphocytes. Contamination, a significant problem in cell culture, requires efforts to prevent it. Certainly the addition of antibiotics will help, but the student must maintain aseptic technique.

## SELECTED REFERENCES

Click, R. E., L. Benck, and B. J. Alter. 1972. Enhancement of antibody synthesis in vitro by mercaptoethanol. *Cell. Imm.* 3:156.

deDuve, C., and H. Beaufay. 1981. A short history of tissue fractionation. *J. Cell Biol.* 91:293.

Freshney, R. I. 1993. *Culture of animal cells. A manual of basic techniques.* 3d ed. New York, NY: Wiley-Liss.

Freshney, R. I., ed. 1992. *Animal cell culture.* 2d ed. New York, NY: IRL Press at Oxford University Press.

Ham, R. G. 1965. Clonal growth of mammalian cells in a chemically defined, synthetic medium. *Proc. Natl. Acad. Sci.* 53:288.

Mishell, R. I., and R. W. Dutton. 1966. Immunization of normal mouse cell suspensions in vitro. *Science.* 153:1004.

# *Identification of B Lymphocytes*

## INTRODUCTION

Lymphocytes are produced in the bone marrow and migrate to the thymus and other tissues where they play important roles in the immune process. All lymphocytes do not exhibit the same properties, especially surface properties. Because of this, lymphocytes can be identified as either B or T by probing for specific **surface markers** characteristic of the B or T lymphocyte. In the mouse, for example, B cells make up from 5 to 15% of the circulating lymphocytes and are identified as such by the presence of antibody molecules (markers) inserted into the membrane. T cells in the mouse contain different antigenic surface markers.

Both B and T cell markers can be recognized by several techniques. Fluorescent monoclonal antibody probes used in conjunction with flow cytometry allow the investigator to separate B and T cells on the basis of both fluorescence and size and are used extensively in research and in the clinical setting. This approach provides the basis for the study of subpopulations of lymphocytes and the unique activities associated with each population.

This exercise involves a procedure designed specifically for the **study of B cells.** It uses a fluorescent dye conjugated to antibodies that detect **surface immunoglobulin** (sIg) on B cells. Most B cells produce and express both IgM and IgD antibodies which can be detected with fluresceinated anti-IgM or anti-IgD. Following the treatment of cells with fluorescein-conjugated antibodies, B cells can be differentiated from T cells by specific fluorescence seen through an ultraviolet (fluorescence) microscope with appropriate filters (figure 16.1).

Antibodies used to identify B cells are preferably monoclonal with a specificity for antibody on the B cell surface. These conjugate to fluorescein isothiocyanate (FITC). Specificity for the IgM antibody is directed to an isotypic marker called mu found on the heavy chains of the IgM antibody molecule. Those B cells that express sIg of the IgM

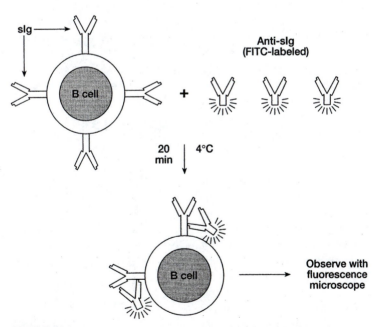

**FIGURE 16.1**
Fluorescent B cells result from interaction of FITC-labeled anti-sIg with sIg. The labeled antibody binds to determinants on heavy chains of sIg and causes B cells to fluoresce.

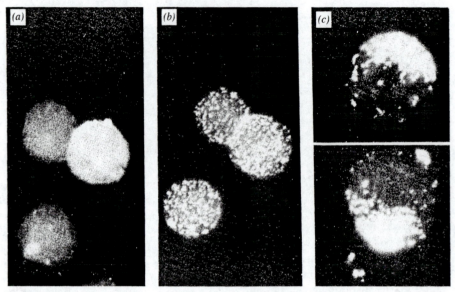

**FIGURE 16.2**

Antibody-induced redistribution of the protein antigen on tumor cells. (*a*) In one experiment (direct staining method), the native distribution of the protein was assessed by fixing the cells first with glutaraldehyde, then staining with fluoresceinated Ig specific for the protein antigens in question. (*b*) In a patching experiment (indirect staining method), the proteins were patched by reacting the cells first with unlabeled IgG specific for the protein antigens in question, then with fluoresceinated anti-IgG, all steps in the presence of sodium azide. (*c*) In a final related experiment, the proteins can be capped at 37° C by omitting the sodium azide in the procedure described in (*b*).

Source: *The Experimental Foundations of Modern Immunology,* third edition. William R. Clark, figure 4.18, page 124. Copyright © 1980 by John Wiley & Sons, Inc. Publishers. Reprinted by permission of Wiley.

type will be detected in this exercise by a fluorescein-tagged, anti-IgM antibody which binds to mu.

Consequences of binding of antibody to membrane-bound antibody on B cells are phenomena known as *patching* and *capping*. Antibodies, as well as certain other agents, cross-link sIg. Some membrane proteins, sIg particularly, are mobile in the cell membrane, and as a result, cross-linking of sIg produces visible patches of **precipitated sIg.** Redistribution of the sIg to one pole of the cell follows patching. Eventually, migration into a polar cap (capping) is complete, and the cell either sheds or ingests the cap (figure 16.2). Capping may lead to B cell proliferation and antibody secretion.

This exercise demonstrates the presence of surface immunoglobulin (sIgM) on B cells isolated from rabbits. It uses a direct staining method that allows observation of the distribution of sIgM. Fluorochrome-labeled (fluorescein isothiocyanate) anti-IgM will be added directly to rabbit lymphocytes and after an incubation period (for the antibodies to react with sIgM), the cells will be observed for fluorescence.

In an alternative method, unlabeled anti-IgM is added to lymphocytes, the excess removed, and a fluorochrome-labeled antibody to the unlabeled anti-IgM is added. The method is referred to as the "sandwich" or indirect technique. The **indirect fluorescent antibody test** can measure either antigen or antibody, including the detection of anti-

gens on tissue sections that have bound antibodies. The antibody can be detected with fluorescent-labeled antibody (antiglobulin serum).

This exercise as written demonstrates patching but not capping. The 4° C incubation temperature slows metabolic activity of the lymphocytes, and this inhibits capping. Additionally, sodium azide, added to the medium, chemically prohibits metabolic activity to further inhibit capping.

## MATERIALS

(Per pair)

HEPES-buffered balanced salt solution (HEPES-BSS)

Histopaque-1077 (Sigma, St. Louis, MO)

Heparin

2 15-ml centrifuge tubes

12-ml syringe with 18-gauge, 2-inch needle

70% ethyl alcohol

5-ml pipettes (sterile)

1-ml pipettes (sterile)

Capillary pipettes (sterile)

Hemacytometer

Centrifuge tubes (12 × 75-mm tubes)

FITC labeled-anti-rabbit IgM (mu chain specific)

Ice

Micropipettes (50 μl)

Mounting medium (e. g., Fluoromount-G, Fisher
Scientific, Pittsburgh, PA)

Coverslips

Microscope slides

UV (fluorescence) microscope

Fetal calf serum (FCS)

Glassware for buffer preparation

Filter for sterilization of media

Tubes for dilution series

(Per class)

1 rabbit

## PROCEDURE

1. Prepare HEPES-buffered balanced salt solution
   (HEPES-BSS) for the isolation and manipulation
   of cells, as described in the appendix. Hanks'
   balanced salt solution or a culture medium such
   as RPMI 1640 that has been supplemented with
   fetal calf serum also provides good results.
2. Collect blood from an anesthetized rabbit as
   described in exercise 1. Each pair of students
   will need 3 ml of blood. Blood from other
   species (including humans) may be substituted if
   the appropriate antiserum is available. Use
   heparin to prevent clotting.
3. Add 5 ml of HEPES-BSS to 3 ml of heparinized
   rabbit blood and mix.
4. Dispense 3.0 ml of a cell separation medium
   such as Histopaque-1077 into a 15-ml centrifuge
   tube. Histopaque-1077 has a density of 1.077 to
   facilitate separation of viable lymphocytes from
   blood by density centrifugation.
5. Carefully, **layer** the diluted blood sample over
   the separation medium. Centrifuge at 400 × g
   for exactly 30 min at room temperature. The use
   of a **swinging bucket rotor** provides the best
   results.
6. Notice the **opaque interface** that results from
   centrifugation. This contains the mononuclear
   cells (figure 16.3). Carefully remove the upper
   layer with a capillary pipette to within 0.5 cm of
   the mononuclear cell layer. Discard the upper
   layer.
7. Remove the opaque interface with a capillary
   pipette and dispense into another 15-ml tube.
   Add 10 ml of HEPES-BSS to the tube and mix
   gently.

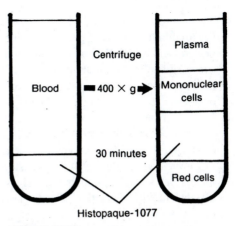

**FIGURE 16.3**
Blood separates into cellular components when
using a separation medium such as Histopaque-
1077. After centrifugation at 400 × g for 30
minutes, the mononuclear cells appear in a
discrete band.
Courtesy Sigma Diagnostics, St. Louis, Missouri.

8. Centrifuge at 250 × g in a swinging bucket rotor
   for 10 min to pellet the cells. (The Eppendorf
   microcentrifuge and tubes can be substituted, but
   use smaller but equivalent volumes). Carefully
   decant and discard the supernatant. The pellet
   will be small (and perhaps difficult to see). Add
   5 ml of HEPES-BSS to resuspend the cells and
   repeat the centrifugation procedure. Be careful
   not to lose cells.
9. After the final centrifugation, add 1 ml of
   HEPES-BSS with 5% FCS, count the cells using
   a hemacytometer, and resuspend to $2 \times 10^6$
   cells/ml using HEPES-BSS with 5% FCS and
   0.2% sodium azide. Centrifuge 1 ml of the cell
   suspension at 250 × g for 10 min.
10. Carefully remove the supernatant from the pellet
    of cells with a capillary pipette. Add 50 μl of
    FITC-labeled-anti-rabbit IgM (mu chain
    specific). **Important:** Check the manufacturer's
    instructions for dilution of the antiserum to make
    a workable dilution. Resuspend the cells in the
    antiserum by mixing gently.
11. Incubate on ice for 20 min. Gently mix two or
    three times during the incubation period.
12. After the incubation period, centrifuge the cells
    at 250 × g to once again pellet the cells. Remove
    the supernatant and discard. Resuspend the cells
    in 1 ml of HEPES-BSS with 5% FCS and once
    again centrifuge. Repeat this procedure 2 more
    times to remove fluorescent material not attached
    to the cells.

13. Place a drop of mounting medium such as Fluoromount-G (Fisher Scientific) or 90% glycerol in HEPES-BSS on a clean microscope slide. Add a drop of the stained cells to the mounting medium. Carefully place a coverslip over the cells (do not trap air bubbles).

14. Observe using a UV (fluorescence) microscope with appropriate filters to allow visualization of cells tagged with FITC-labeled antibodies. Use a magnification of 400 to 500X (some students may prefer 1000X oil immersion). The slides may be stored in the dark at 4° C for later observation.

15. Determine the percentage of B lymphocytes. Do this by first counting the number of lymphocytes in a field with normal light. Make certain to count only lymphocytes, which are small, round cells with little cytoplasm. After counting the total number of lymphocytes, count the fluorescent cells in the same field with UV light and determine the percent of B cells by dividing the number of fluorescent cells by the total lymphocytes and multiplying by 100.

## DISCUSSION

Since the assay for sIg as described works equally well for all species, the instructor may decide to use human lymphocytes or lymphocytes from a species other than the rabbit. Keep in mind, however, that the anti-IgM antibodies must be specific for the species used. Also, remember that this exercise can be extended to demonstrate capping. Since capping requires metabolic activity, the extended procedure should be done at 37° C instead of on ice.

Occasionally, nonspecific staining occurs. This may be due to an excess of labeled antibody. Check the manufacturer's instructions for dilution or, if the labeled antibody has been produced in-house, titer the antisera to determine the optimum dilution to provide the desired results.

When counting fluorescent cells, it is best not to count those that have a uniform fluorescence; these cells are probably dead. Explain. Realizing that some cells will die, the student may want to do a viability study. This may be accomplished using the Trypan Blue exclusion method discussed in exercise 15. A good slide preparation should have approximately 30 cells per field, but remember that all cells isolated with the separation medium are not B cells. Those that are not should not fluoresce and can serve as non-B cell or **non-fluorescent controls.**

The problems that usually occur with this technique result from: (1) the inability of the student to recognize lymphocytes and perhaps identify fluorescent cells, (2) difficulties in lymphocyte preparation, and (3) reagent problems that might cause nonspecific immunofluorescence. HEPES-BSS with 5% FCS is suggested for this exercise to maintain or even enhance viability, but a medium such as RPMI 1640 with 5% FCS will perform as well.

An alternative to the wet mount preparation described in this exercise is a dry mount of the fluorescent cells. Prepare it by allowing the cells to dry on the microscope slide, then fix them for 20 sec with 95% ethyl alcohol. When dry, add a drop of mounting fluid and a coverslip and view microscopically. A procedure is also available for dry mounts using 1% paraformaldehyde.

## SELECTED REFERENCES

Baum, C. M., J. M. Davie, and J. P. McKearn. 1985. B-Cell subsets: functional and structural characteristics. *CRC Crit. Rev. Immunol.* 5:349.

Beutner, E. H., R. J. Nisengard, and B. Allini, eds. 1983. Defined immunofluorescence and related cytochemical methods. *Ann. N.Y. Acad. Sci.* 420:1.

Bullock, G., ed. 1984. *Techniques in immunochemistry.* Orlando, FL: Academic Press, Inc.

Cambier, J. C., J. G. Monroe, K. M. Coggeshall, and J. T. Ransom. 1985. The biochemical basis of transmembrane signalling by B lymphocyte surface immunoglobulin. *Immunol. Today.* 6:218.

Mills, G. B., ed. 1993. Transmembrane signaling through hematopoietin receptors: interleukin-2 and erythropoietin. In *Seminars in immunology.* 5:5.

Moller, G. 1961. Demonstration of mouse isoantigens at the cellular level by the fluorescent antibody technique. *J. Exp. Med.* 114:415.

Moller, G., ed. 1983. B cell differentiation antigens. *Immunol. Rev.* 69:5.

Raff, M. C., M. Sternberg, and R. B. Taylor. 1970. Immunoglobulin determinants on the surface of mouse lymphoid cells. *Nature.* 225:553.

Sternberger, L. A. 1986. *Immunocytochemistry.* 3d ed. New York, NY: John Wiley and Sons, Inc.

Zola, H. 1987. The surface antigens of human B lymphocytes. *Immunol. Today.* 8(10):308.

# 17

# *Identification of T Lymphocytes*

## INTRODUCTION

**T lymphocytes** serve as important components of the cell-mediated immune response, and frequently require identification. More than 70% of peripheral blood lymphocytes are T cells. These cells play an important role in defense against infections caused by intracellular agents such as viruses, some bacteria, fungi, and protozoa. When T cells are stimulated by antigen, they may become cytotoxic to those cells expressing the antigen, and, in addition, may produce lymphokines that have an overall stimulatory effect on immune defense against infectious disease.

T cell identification is important because of the clinical relevance of T cell numbers. For example, T cell numbers decrease in older individuals, and some authorities suggest that the decrease may have some bearing on the higher incidence of carcinoma in the older age groups. Tests for T cell numbers, therefore, provide information about impairment of **cell-mediated immunity.**

Two reliable methods can identify human T cells. One popular method uses **monoclonal antibodies** that have been specifically produced to react with a variety of surface antigens that are unique to the various subpopulations of T cells. The monoclonal antibodies can be tagged with fluorochrome to verify the reaction.

The other method used to identify (and enumerate) T cells is the **sheep erythrocyte (E) rosette test.** T cells isolated from human peripheral blood can bind sheep erythrocytes via the CD2 receptor on T cells and consequently form a rosette. T cell receptors that bind to determinants on the sheep cells do so in a nonimmune manner (figure 17.1). The T cell appears within the cluster of sheep erythrocytes. This method provides a convenient way to separate T cells from B cells for **identification and enumeration.**

This exercise directs the student through: (1) a procedure for the separation of T cells from human peripheral blood, and (2) the rosette assay for the determination of the percentage of T cells in blood. In brief, peripheral blood mononuclear cells are first isolated with density centrifugation, and then sheep erythrocytes are added. The preparation is viewed microscopically, and lymphocytes that have

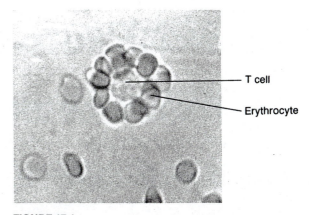

**FIGURE 17.1**
An E rosette formed when sheep erythrocytes are mixed with T cells. The erythrocytes bind to the surface of the T cells, resulting in aggregate formation with a T cell found within a cluster of SRBC.

three or more erythrocytes adhering to their surface are considered to be T cells.

Since this exercise requires the use of human blood, students should consider the potential hazards associated with the study of blood. The student should realize that laboratory animals work nicely for the study of most immunological phenomena in a beginning immunology course. However, significant differences exist between animal immune systems and human immune systems, and the study of animal models do not fully apply to the human in all cases. This exercise focuses on a specific trait of **human T cells.**

When a laboratory study focuses on the human immune system, the student must realize the associated risks of infection with disease agents such as the HIV-1, hepatitis B virus, other viruses, and bacterial agents as discussed in exercise 3. To prevent laboratory-acquired infections, the following safety rules should be strictly enforced: (1) decontaminate work areas, especially surfaces, before and after work; (2) do not eat or drink in the laboratory; (3) wear a laboratory coat or smock; (4) do not mouth pipette; (5) wash hands frequently; (6) work in a biosafety cabinet; and (7) autoclave all waste materials.

## MATERIALS

(Per pair)

HEPES-buffered balanced salt solution (HEPES-
  BSS) with and without 5% fetal calf serum (FCS)

Sheep red blood cells (SRBC)

3 ml human blood

Capillary pipettes

1-ml pipettes

5-ml pipettes

Hemacytometer

Heparin

Needle and syringe or Vacutainer® for venipuncture

Tourniquet

Alcohol swabs

12 × 75-mm tube

Histopaque-1077 (Sigma, St. Louis, MO)

15-ml centrifuge tubes

Trypan Blue solution

## PROCEDURE

1. Prepare a solution of HEPES-buffered balanced salt solution (HEPES-BSS) with and without 5% fetal calf serum (FCS). See the appendix for formulations.

2. Prepare a suspension of fresh sheep red blood cells (SRBC) by diluting 1 part cells in 4 parts HEPES-BSS. Gently mix and centrifuge at 200 × g for 5 min to pellet the cells. Remove the supernatant and discard. Repeat this procedure and resuspend the cells in HEPES-BSS with 5% FCS. Count the cells using a hemacytometer and dilute to $4 \times 10^8$ SRBC/ml in HEPES-BSS with 5% FCS. Include dilution factors when calculating cells/ml from the hemacytometer count. Set aside until needed.

3. Have a qualified individual withdraw 3 ml of blood into heparin (0.1 mg/ml) using the venipuncture procedure demonstrated by the instructor and used in exercise 1. Be sure to read the comments presented in the introduction to this exercise and follow the rules for safety in the laboratory. Alternatively, your instructor may provide you with a sample of human blood.

4. Add 5 ml of HEPES-BSS with 5% FCS to the heparinized blood and mix.

5. Repeat steps 4 through 8 of exercise 16 to produce a suspension of human mononuclear cells. However, wash the cells each time with HEPES-BSS plus 5% FCS. Use a swinging bucket rotor in the centrifuge and be especially careful when decanting supernatant so that the pelleted cells are not discarded.

6. Add 1 ml of HEPES-BSS with FCS and gently mix. Make dilutions to obtain the appropriate number of cells for counting and count the cells using a hemacytometer. Prepare a final suspension of $1 \times 10^7$ cells/ml.

7. Pipette 0.5 ml of the lymphocyte suspension into a 12 × 75-mm tube. Pipette 0.5 ml of the SRBC suspension prepared in step 2 into the same tube and gently mix.

8. Centrifuge at 250 × g for 5 min. Remove the centrifuge tube carefully so that the cells are not disturbed and incubate at room temperature for 1.5 to 2 hr.

9. After the incubation period, very carefully resuspend the cells (and rosettes) by gently tilting the tube back and forth. Add 0.1 ml of Trypan Blue solution and once again gently mix the cells. The Trypan Blue procedure as described in exercise 15 will help the student distinguish living from dead cells.

10. With a capillary pipette, **gently transfer** the rosettes to a clean microscope slide and add a coverslip. Place the coverslip over the rosettes so that no air bubbles form. Observe the rosettes using the 40X objective.

11. Count only those lymphocytes that are surrounded by three or more SRBC. Record the number. Determine the total number of lymphocytes (count at least 200 lymphocytes) and calculate the percentage of T lymphocytes in human blood by dividing the number of lymphocytes in rosettes by the number of lymphocytes in rosettes **plus** the number not in rosettes and multiply by 100.

## DISCUSSION

Take care to distinguish lymphocytes from sheep red blood cells. These cells are approximately the same size, but the lymphocytes are not as round as red cells and are also refractile because of the nucleus.

Although more can be learned about the mechanism of T cell binding to red blood cells, the E receptor has been determined to be a polypeptide with a molecular weight of around 50,000. In mice it is called the CD2 (Leu5) receptor.

The procedure relies heavily upon careful centrifugation and resuspension of the fragile rosettes. The final centrifugation step assures close proximity of T cells to form the E rosette. Some investigators prefer to incubate overnight at 4° C.

The rosette procedure can be expanded and used as a method for isolation of T cells by separating T cells from bound SRBC by hypotonic lysis of the SRBC. The population obtained with this procedure contains greater than 95% T cells.

A suggested extension of the procedure uses neuraminidase-treated SRBC to enhance binding of the SRBC to T cells. The protocol requires the incubation of washed SRBC in neuraminidase for 1 hr at 37° C.

## SELECTED REFERENCES

*Biosafety in microbiological and biomedical laboratories.* Health and Human Services Publication (NIH) 88-8395. Washington, DC: U.S. Government Printing Office.

Cantor, H., and E. A. Boyse. 1975. Functional subclasses of T lymphocytes bearing different Ly antigens. I: The generation of functionally distinct T cell subclasses is a differentiative process independent of antigen. *J. Exp. Med.* 141:1375.

Kronenberg, M. G., G. Siu, L. E. Hood, and N. Shastri. 1986. The molecular generation of the T-cell antigen receptor and T-antigen recognition. *Ann. Rev. Immunol.* 4:529.

Marrack, P., and J. Kappler. 1987. The T cell receptor. *Science.* 238:1073.

Parish, C. R., S. M. Kirov, N. Bowern, and R. V. Blanden. 1974. A one-step procedure for separating mouse T and B lymphocytes. *Eur. J. Immunol.* 4:808.

Weiner, M. S., C. Bianco, and V. Nussenzweig. 1973. Enhanced binding of neuraminidase-treated sheep erythrocytes to human T lymphocytes. *Blood.* 42:939.

# Lymphocyte Response to Mitogens

## INTRODUCTION

Both B and T lymphocytes respond when influenced by substances called **mitogens.** A number of mitogens used in immunology have different chemical characteristics, but all have the ability to induce lymphocytes to enter mitosis (thus the name mitogen). Mitogens are used extensively in the study of cellular immunology, and the discovery of many fundamental cellular mechanisms can be attributed to their use.

Mitogens can substitute for antigens to induce mitosis and initiate lymphocyte proliferation. Treatment with mitogens elicits a proliferative (blastogenic) response in a large percentage of the cell population and this serves as **polyclonal activators.** Some mitogens stimulate only B cells; others only T cells. It appears that mitogens interact with carbohydrate groups (glycoproteins) on the surface of all lymphocytes but yet may be specific for B or T cells. As an example, **Phytohemagglutinin** and **Concanavalin A** are lectins (plant proteins or glycoproteins) that stimulate subpopulations of T cells. **Pokeweed mitogen** causes the proliferation of both T and B lymphocytes, and lipopolysaccharide stimulates only B cells (of rodents). Table 18.1 lists selected mitogens commonly used in both clinical and research immunology and some characteristics of each.

The lymphocyte response to mitogens is nonspecific, whereas the response to antigens (also mitosis-stimulating agents) is specific. Particular antigens stimulate only a small number of lymphocytes, but nonimmunogenic substances like mitogens cause large numbers of cells to transform. Antigens in vitro stimulate lymphocytes from **sensitized donors** only, but mitogens stimulate lymphocytes without presensitization of the donor. Stimulation by specific and nonspecific activators apparently causes the same biochemical events. Figure 18.1 shows the response of immature T cells sensitized by antigen-presenting cells, alloantigen, or mitogen and illustrates one useful method to detect cellular proliferation that follows stimulation. The cellular events that occur after sensitization of an immature lymphocyte are called **lymphocyte transformation.** The resulting cells can influence immune reactions and may be referred to as effector cells.

DNA synthesis has been used as the basis for many assay methods that determine the response of lymphocytes to activators because DNA synthesis correlates well with cell growth. In most methods, **DNA synthesis** is measured by the incorporation of $^3$H-thymidine into nuclear material. Uptake of $^3$H-thymidine by stimulated cells is compared to uptake by control cells that have not been stimulated.

This exercise demonstrates the response of splenic lymphocytes to **nonspecific activators.** Murine spleen cells will be stimulated with Concanavalin A (Con A) in the presence of $^3$H-thymidine and other DNA precursors. This results in a blastogenic T cell response, indicated by an increase in DNA synthesis as measured by the uptake of $^3$H-thymidine. This is the first of two exercises that requires the **use of a tritium compound.** Students should listen carefully to directions for the proper use of radioisotopes; these exercises may require licensure for the use of radioisotopes.

**Table 18.1** Selected Mitogens

| Mitogen | Source | Molecular Weight | Cells Stimulated |
|---|---|---|---|
| Concanavalin A (ConA) | *Canavalia einsformis* | 55,000 | T (human and mouse) |
| Phytohemagglutinin (PHA) | *Phaseolus vulgaris* | 140,000 | T (human and mouse) |
| Pokeweed mitogen (PWM) | *Phytolacca americana* | 32,000 | T and B |
| Lipopolysaccharide (LPS) | Gram—negative bacteria | 1,000,000 to 24,000,000 | B (mouse) |
| Dextran sulfate | — | 500,000 | B |

Useful in microgram/ml quantities.

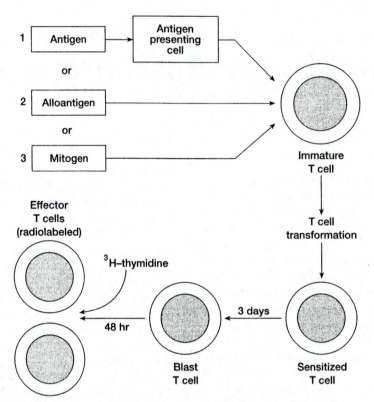

**FIGURE 18.1**

T cell proliferation in response to stimuli. The resting T cell can be stimulated to transform by antigen or mitogen. Transformation involves proliferation and, consequently, DNA synthesis. The thymidine required for DNA synthesis has been labeled with $^3$H. The result is a tag on the effector T cells produced as a result of T cell stimulation.

## MATERIALS

(Per pair)

1 mouse

Hemacytometer and coverslip

Sterile capillary pipettes

1-ml pipettes

5-ml pipettes

Sterile 15-ml centrifuge tubes

Centrifuge

RPMI 1640 plus 5% fetal calf serum (FCS) and supplemented with 100 U/ml penicillin and 100 μg/ml streptomycin

12 × 100-mm cell culture tubes

12 × 75-mm cell culture tubes with caps

Concanavalin A (Con A)

Trypan Blue solution

$^3$H-thymidine (ICN Radiochemicals, Irvine, CA)

Filters (0.45 μ pore size) and filter holders (Millipore Corp., Bedford, MA)

Trichloroacetic acid (TCA) (10% solution)

Ethyl alcohol (95%)

Scintillation vials

Scintillation fluid

Scintillation counter

Tris-buffered ammonium chloride

$CO_2$ for mouse euthanasia

Plastic Petri dish

Surgical instruments (scalpel, scissors, forceps)

Rubber policeman

Glassware for media and buffer preparation

$CO_2$ incubator (37° C)

## PROCEDURE

1. Successful completion of this exercise requires accurate pipetting, aseptic technique and proper dilution and addition of isotope.

2. Prepare isotonic Tris-buffered ammonium chloride to lyse red blood cells found in the spleen cell suspension. Use the procedure in the appendix to prepare the ammonium chloride.

3. A stock solution of Con A in RPMI 1640 should be prepared. The exact dilution of this mitogen must be calculated for each lot of Con A purchased, but a good starting point for this exercise would be 0.1 ml of Con A solution into 1 ml of cells to give a final concentration of approximately 5 μg of Con A/ml of cells.

4. Prepare a spleen cell suspension as outlined in steps 1 through 8 of exercise 15. However, for this exercise use RPMI 1640 supplemented with 5% FCS, 100 U/ml penicillin and 100 μg/ml streptomycin.

5. Centrifuge the cells at $250 \times g$ for 10 min and resuspend in 2 ml of the isotonic Tris-buffered ammonium chloride solution. Incubate for 2 min at 37° C.

6. Carefully add 2 ml of FCS **under the suspended cells** (why?) with a capillary pipette and centrifuge at $250 \times g$ for 10 min.

7. Discard the supernatant and wash the cells 2 times with medium.

8. After the final wash, resuspend the cells in 1 ml warm RPMI 1640 with 5% FCS and count with a hemacytometer. Dilute to $1 \times 10^6$ cells/ml. Each pair of students will need at least 7 ml of suspended cells. These cells will be assayed for Con A induction of a T cell **blastogenic response.**

9. Add 1 ml of the $1 \times 10^6$ cell suspension to each of 6, $12 \times 75$-ml cell culture tubes and cap them.

10. Add 0.1 ml of the Con A solution (stock solution) from step 3 to three tubes of cells. Label them "experimental." Add 0.1 ml of media to the other three tubes. Label them "control." Loosely cap all tubes. If desired, another tube can be prepared for Trypan Blue viability determinations.

11. Incubate all of the tubes in a 37° C, 5% $CO_2$, humidified incubator for 3 da. Do not disturb the tubes. However, check periodically for microbial contamination and discard contaminated tubes.

12. After the incubation period, add 0.1 ml of medium containing 10 microCi/ml $^3$H-thymidine to each of the experimental and control tubes. The preparation of diluted isotope will vary depending upon the **specific activity** of the material received from the supplier. This step may require the use of a specially designed radioisotope facility. Be sure to follow rules and regulations provided by the instructor regarding the safe handling and use of radioisotopes.

13. Incubate for 48 hr under the conditions described in step 11.

14. In the meantime, set up a filtration system that uses a filter with a 0.45 μ pore size that is suitable for radiochemical assays. The radiolabeled cells will be trapped on the filter.

15. Pour the cells (and culture medium) from each of the six tubes onto separate filters. Apply suction. Wash each culture tube with 2 ml of medium and pour onto the appropriate filter. Repeat two times. Take care not to lose labeled cells.

16. Next, lyse the cells on each filter and remove TCA-soluble materials by adding 10 ml of a cold 10% TCA solution. Suction through the filter. Repeat this procedure.

17. Wash the TCA insoluble precipitate that remains on the filter with 5 ml of 95% ethyl alcohol. Repeat two times.

18. Place each filter in a separate scintillation vial. Label appropriately.

19. Place all scintillation vials in a 37° C incubator overnight (with caps removed) to dry. Make certain that the filters are **completely dry** before proceeding.

20. Add 5 ml of **scintillation fluid** provided by the instructor to each vial. This step should cause the filters to become transparent.

21. Determine counts per minute (cpm) in an appropriate scintillation counter using directions for use of the instrument supplied by the instructor.

22. Calculate the stimulation index (SI) by dividing the mean cpm of experimental samples (with mitogen) by the mean cpm of the control sample (without mitogen).

## DISCUSSION

Although an exact amount of mitogen has been suggested, keep in mind that the supplier may provide shipments of mitogens that differ from other shipments received from the same source. For this reason, test each lot of mitogen to determine the amount necessary to cause the maximal cell response. Use the recommendations given in this exercise as a starting point. Optimum conditions for each assay are empirical and should be established by the student.

Tritiated thymidine can be purchased from a variety of suppliers. Purchase a product that will have a specific activity (e.g., 2 Ci/mmol) that will give an appropriate final dilution. Remember that students must follow the institution's rules and regulations regarding the safe handling and use of radiochemicals. However, shielding is not required because $^3$H produces low-energy β particles.

The described procedures can be altered to enhance speed and accuracy. Such an alteration involves the use of **microtiter plates** and a **cell harvester.**

Finally, cell proliferation studies have a number of applications in a clinical setting. For example, an individual's lymphocyte response to a specific antigen as determined by a proliferative assay as outlined in this exercise may indicate immunologic suppression and, therefore, an immune defect.

## SELECTED REFERENCES

Evans, E. A. 1974. *Tritium and its compounds.* New York, NY: Wiley.

Hendke, W. R. 1973. *Radioactive tracings in biological research.* New York, NY: Wiley.

Jannosy, G., and M. F. Greaves. 1972. Lymphocyte activation. I. Response of T and B lymphocytes to phytomitogens. *Clin. Exp. Immunol.* 9:483.

Oppenheim, J. J., and D. L. Rosenstreich. 1976. *Mitogens in immunobiology.* New York, NY: Academic Press.

Strong, D. M., A. A. Ahmed, G. B. Thurman, and K. W. Sell. 1973. In vitro stimulation of murine spleen cells using a microculture system and a multiple automated sample harvester. *J. Immunol. Meth.* 2:279.

# Cellular Communication

## INTRODUCTION

Cells of the immune system resemble other mammalian cells in a number of ways. Like other cells, immune cells communicate with each other; this ability contributes significantly to the reliability of the immune system. A significant part of this communication is mediated by a group of **soluble cell factors** that function much like hormones. Some of these factors, produced by lymphocytes, are appropriately called **lymphokines;** macrophages (and monocytes) produce soluble mediator molecules called **monokines.** Collectively, immune system regulatory molecules are called **cytokines.** All of these factors provide information to a variety of cells.

It was once believed that B and T cells, as well as macrophages, interacted directly with all antigens without the intervention of soluble mediators. We now know that many cellular immune functions involve cytokines. The cytokines play a particularly important role as immunopotentiating and immunoregulatory mediators, and although many of them have been discovered and characterized, there are probably others as yet unidentified. Table 19.1 lists those that are important for immunologic competence.

One of the first identified lymphokines was **migration inhibition factor** (MIF). Initially shown to be present in spleen cell culture supernatant generated in vitro by splenocytes and antigens, MIF inhibited the migration of macrophages. Later, researchers discovered that lymphocytes sensitized to antigen produce MIF and direct it to a more or less passive target cell, the macrophage. As a consequence of a MIF-target cell interaction, the macrophage becomes activated.

Conversely, the macrophage functions as an accessory cell and produces products responsible for the activation of lymphocytes. One of the first lymphocyte activators to be discovered was a substance that caused proliferation of thymocytes in the presence of the mitogen, Concanavalin A. Thymocytes are pre-T cells that originate in the bone marrow and migrate to the thymus. The substance that causes proliferation of them was appropriately named **lymphocyte-activating factor** (LAF). Other names have been proposed, and it is now called **interleukin-1** (IL-1). This name describes its ability to mediate communication among leukocytes. Another factor produced by T cells also plays an obligatory role in promoting long-term growth of cytotoxic T lymphocytes. Originally named T-cell growth factor (TCGF), it has been renamed **interleukin-2** (IL-2). Many other interleukins have been discovered and reported. These products can be induced in vitro by a variety of different stimulating agents.

Monokines and lymphokines act in concert to initiate and maintain the immune cascade. In many cases interaction of immune cells requires the participation of several factors. For example, IL-1 and IL-2 cause **antigen specific**

**Table 19.1** Some Important Cytokines

| Cytokine | Source | Function |
|---|---|---|
| Interleukin 1 (IL-1) or lymphocyte activating factor | Macrophage | T cell mitogenesis and production of IL-2 |
| Interleukin 2 (IL-2) or T cell growth factor | Lymphocyte | T cell mitogenesis |
| B cell growth factor (BCGF) | Mononuclear cell and lymphocyte | B cell mitogenesis |
| Granulocyte-macrophage colony-stimulating factor (GM-CSF) | T cell, monocyte, and other mammalian cells | Control maturation, differentiation, and proliferation |
| Tumor necrosis factor (TNF) | Macrophage and lymphocyte | Inhibit growth and cytotoxic for tumors |
| Lymphotoxin (LT) | Macrophage, lymphocyte, and natural killer cell | Inhibit growth and cytotoxic for cells |

These molecules serve as chemical messengers between sets of immune cells.

**T cell activation and proliferation.** The sequence of events follows: IL-1 is produced and released by antigen-presenting macrophages. The macrophage interacts with receptors on a resting CD4$^+$ T cell (figure 19.1) in an MHC-restricted manner. This interaction is necessary for the CD4$^+$ T cell to become fully activated to antigen presented by the macrophage. As a consequence of activation, the T cells produce IL-2 (in addition to a variety of other lymphokines) and the receptors for it. Interaction of IL-2 with these receptors induces T cell proliferation. Figure 19.2 depicts this series of activities. IL-2 is also necessary for pre-cytotoxic T cells to recognize and become activated by macrophage-bound antigen.

Exercise 19 is designed as an assay for IL-1 activity. Cultured macrophages will be stimulated to produce this cytokine. When it is released into the cell culture supernatant, it will diffuse through a semipermeable membrane to interact with thymocytes that have been treated with phytohemagglutinin (PHA). The assay is commonly called a **thymocyte comitogenic assay.** The exercise demonstrates the existence of molecules which act as mediators for an appropriate interaction of immune cells.

The exercise involves, first of all, the isolation of murine peritoneal macrophages and stimulation of them with lipopolysaccharide (LPS) to produce IL-1. Secondly, a population of cells (thymocytes) will be isolated and briefly exposed to the mitogen, PHA, to stimulate transformation. The stimulated thymocytes will be placed in one chamber of a Marbrook vessel, and LPS-stimulated macrophages will be placed in the other chamber. These will be separated from one another by only a semipermeable membrane. Upon incubation, macrophages will produce soluble IL-1 that will pass through the membrane and cause thymocytes to proliferate. IL-1 activity will be determined by measuring **thymocyte proliferation.**

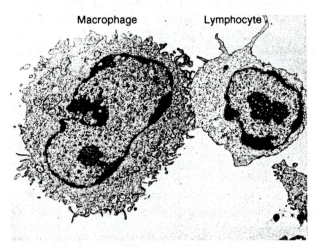

**FIGURE 19.1**

An electron photomicrograph showing a macrophage (left) and a lymphocyte (right). These cells are in contact with each other, a situation that is not unusual. This interaction of the T cell with the HLA class-II MHC molecules on the surface of the macrophage is required for a helper T cell to respond to some antigens.

Source: Rosenthal, Alan S. *New England Journal of Medicine* 303(1980): 1153.

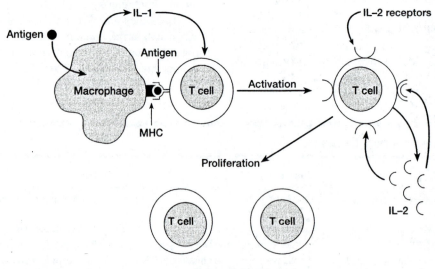

**FIGURE 19.2**

The role of interleukin in the T cell response to antigen. Small resting T lymphocytes have a single receptor for antigen and MHC determinants. The histocompatible macrophage presents antigen to the T cell to initiate activation; this also requires IL-1. IL-1 is produced by the macrophage (antigen presenting cell). Activation causes the T cell to begin to produce IL-2 and receptors for it. IL-2 is bound to these receptors and replication is initiated to produce a clone of T cells.

From E. S. Golub, *Immunology: A Synthesis* (1987).

## MATERIALS

(Per pair)

2 Marbrook culture vessels (Bellco Glass, Inc., Vineland, NJ)

Membrane filters (0.2 μ porosity) (Millipore Corp., Bedford, MA)

Saline

Distilled water

Swinny adapter (Millipore Corp., Bedford, MA)

10-ml syringes

HEPES-buffered balanced salt solution (HEPES-BSS)

Pipettes

Surgical instruments

Glassware

Capillary pipettes

RPMI 1640 culture medium

Fetal calf serum (FCS)

Mice (any species) for macrophages

Mice (six-week-old C3H/HeJ) for thymocytes (Jackson Laboratories, Bar Harbor, ME)

Mineral oil, sterile

Lipopolysaccharide (LPS)

$CO_2$ incubator

India ink

$CO_2$ for mouse euthanasia

Sterile Petri dishes

Sterile centrifuge tubes

Centrifuge

Hemacytometer

2-mercaptoethanol

Phytohemagglutinin (PHA)

Trypan Blue dye

[3]H-thymidine (New England Nuclear, Boston, MA)

Scintillation counter

Heparin

## PROCEDURE

### Culture Vessel Preparation

1. Prepare Marbrook culture vessels as described in the following steps. Complete this preparation and store the vessels prior to the laboratory period when cells are to be cultured. Figure 19.3 illustrates the Marbrook vessel and its dimensions. The vessel is composed of an upper and lower chamber, and thymocytes and macrophages will be cultured in these

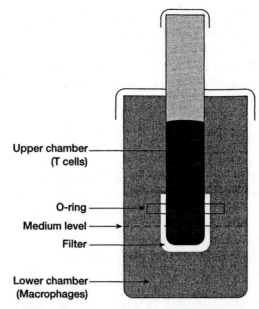

**FIGURE 19.3**
The Marbrook vessel. Macrophages are put into the lower chamber, thymocytes into the upper chamber, with the chambers separated by a semipermeable membrane. The macrophages produce soluble cytokines, which diffuse across the membrane, and thymocytes that have been stimulated with mitogen proliferate.

respectively. Cells will be separated from each other by a semipermeable membrane (0.2 μ porosity) secured to the upper chamber by a rubber O-ring. Each pair of students should have 2 vessels, one for **experimental** and one for **control.**

2. Autoclave both the membrane and O-ring first in saline and again in distilled water to remove contaminating materials. Place the membrane in a Swinny adapter attached to a syringe and wash with 10 ml of HEPES-buffered balanced salt solution (HEPES-BSS). Reverse the membrane and repeat with 10 ml distilled water.

3. Carefully secure the washed membrane to the bottom of the upper chamber of the Marbrook culture vessel with an O-ring. Refer to figure 19.3. Trim away the excess above the O-ring. Keep the membrane wet throughout this step.

4. Put the upper chamber with an attached filter into distilled water in a beaker and autoclave to sterilize. Wrap the lower chamber in aluminum foil or brown paper and sterilize in a dry air oven (160 to 170° C for 2 to 3 hr). After sterilization of both parts, remove the water from the upper chamber with a capillary pipette and place the upper chamber in the lower chamber. Store until needed.

5. At least one day before using, place 10 ml of RPMI 1640 medium supplemented with 10% (FCS) in the lower chamber and place in an incubator at 37° C. When ready to use, withdraw the medium with a capillary pipette and add cells as described below.

## Macrophage Collection

6. **Use aseptic technique** when performing the following procedures. Use care when isolating both macrophages and thymocytes for culture. If desired, antibiotics can be added to the culture medium to help prevent contamination (penicillin, 100 U/ml and streptomycin, 100 $\mu$g/ml).

7. This exercise uses **murine peritoneal macrophages** collected from any species. Obtain the peritoneal cells (peritoneal wash) as described in exercise 4. Briefly, the procedure for collecting peritoneal cells consists of killing the mice and injecting 8 ml of prewarmed RPMI 1640 medium containing 10% FCS and 7 SU/ml sodium heparin IP into each mouse. Lavage and withdraw the medium containing macrophages. Discard if red blood cells are present. Wash the cells twice with medium, count, and prepare 20 ml of a suspension of $3 \times 10^6$ cells/ml in RPMI 1640 with 10% FCS. One mouse should produce approximately $1 \times 10^7$ cells. The peritoneal exudate cell (PEC) suspension will contain a significant number of macrophages.

8. Add 10 ml of PEC suspension to the lower chamber of each of two Marbrook culture vessels and incubate at 37° C in a humid $CO_2$ incubator for 60 min. Macrophages will adhere to the glass during this period of time.

9. After incubation, carefully pour off the medium and add 10 ml of RPMI 1640 medium with 10% FCS. Gently swirl and discard. Repeat. Finally, add 10 ml of fresh medium to one vessel (control) and to the other add medium containing 10 $\mu$g/ml lipopolysaccharide (LPS) (experimental).

10. Incubate in a 5% $CO_2$ incubator at 37° C until ready to add thymocytes to the upper chamber.

## Thymocyte Collection and Preparation

11. C3H/HeJ six-week-old mice should be used as a source of thymocytes. This strain has been shown to be LPS-insensitive and IL-1 responsive and at this age each mouse should produce approximately $2 \times 10^8$ thymocytes.

12. To prevent contamination of the thymocyte suspension with lymph node cells from the area of the thymus, inject the mouse interperitoneally (IP) with India ink 30 min prior to killing the mouse. The India ink will collect in the parathymic lymph nodes and make them visible.

13. Avoid contamination of the thymocyte suspension with red blood cells. To help prevent contamination, bleed the mouse from the marginal tail veins or retro-orbital plexus to remove as much blood as possible and then kill the mouse in $CO_2$. Do not use cervical dislocation because it may cause bleeding in the thoracic area and contaminate the thymus cell suspension with red blood cells.

14. Remember to use aseptic technique! Prevent contamination when performing the following procedures: Cut through the ribs and remove the sternum to expose the thoracic area. The thymus is situated just above the heart and is easily recognized as a white, bilobed organ. See figure 15.2 for an indication of the relative position of the thymus to other thoracic organs. Remove the thymus with scissors but be careful to leave the India ink-stained parathymic lymph nodes. Put the thymus in sterile HEPES-BSS in a sterile Petri dish.

15. Carefully remove all remaining lymph nodes and large blood vessels. Use sterile scissors. Rinse the thymus with sterile HEPES-BSS and place it in another Petri dish containing sterile HEPES-BSS.

16. Tease the thymus apart with sterile forceps. Attempt to produce a single-cell suspension by raking the cells away from cell masses. Continue to do this until there are no pieces left.

17. Allow the remaining fragments to settle to the bottom of the Petri dish and carefully pipette the suspended cells into a centrifuge tube. Centrifuge at $250 \times g$ for 10 min to pellet the cells.

18. Wash once with serile HEPES-BSS and finally with RPMI 1640 with 10% FCS. After the final centrifugation, add a small amount of RPMI 1640 with 10% FCS and count the cells using a hemacytometer. Adjust the cell concentration to $1 \times 10^7$ cells/ml in RPMI 1640 with 10% FCS and $5 \times 10^{-5}$M 2-mercaptoethanol.

19. Add purified phytohemagglutinin (PHA) to the thymocyte suspension to a final concentration of 5 $\mu$g/ml to increase the sensitivity of the thymocytes to IL-1. Incubate for 60 min in a humid $CO_2$ incubator at 37° C.

20. After incubation, wash these cells 2 times with 25 ml of medium to remove unbound PHA.

Resuspend the cells, count, and dilute to $1 \times 10^7$ cells/ml. Check these cells for viability with Trypan Blue.

21. Carefully pipette 0.5 ml of the PHA-stimulated cells into the upper chambers of both the control and experimental Marbrook culture vessels. Quickly place the upper chambers in the lower chambers. Only the semipermeable membranes now separate the thymocytes from macrophages in the lower chambers.

22. Incubate in $CO_2$ at 37° C for 72 hr.

## Cell Proliferation Determination

23. At the end of the incubation period, add 15 microCi of $^3$H-thymidine in RPMI 1640 medium with 10% FCS to the upper chamber of both Marbrook culture vessels and incubate for 6 hr.

24. Following this incubation period, proceed to determine $^3$H incorporation into thymocytes as described in steps 14 through 22 of exercise 18.

25. Compare the proliferation response of thymocytes to factors produced by macrophages stimulated with LPS to those not stimulated. Determine the **stimulation indices** by dividing the cpm thymidine incorporated in the experimental by the cpm thymidine incorporated in the control.

## DISCUSSION

IL-1 is not only a product of monocyte/macrophage cell lines but also dendritic cells, neutrophils, fibroblasts, endothelial cells, certain B cell lines, and others. The assay presented here is a modification of the **mouse thymocyte assay** that measures the substitution of soluble IL-1 for the antigen-presenting macrophage. Other methods such as radioimmunoassay also measure IL-1. An assay for IL-1, developed by Kaye and Janeway, uses a murine helper T cell line designated D10.G4.1 that is exceptionally sensitive to IL-1.

This exercise provides the student with a sophisticated procedure to use methods and skills developed in earlier exercises. However, if desired, the procedure can be abbreviated considerably by using recombinant interleukin 1 (rIL-1) to stimulate thymocytes. IL-1 is available commercially in recombinant form (Genzyme Corp., Boston, MA). Briefly, thymocytes are collected as outlined in steps 11 through 20. Pipette 0.1 ml of cells into wells of a microtiter plate and add 0.1 ml of diluted rIL-1 to each well. Prepare a number of dilutions of rIL-1. Incubate in $CO_2$ at 37° C for 42 hr. Add $^3$H and incubate for an additional 6 hr. Harvest and count as described in exercise 18.

Exercise 19 may be used as a measurement of the accessory cell function of macrophages (i.e., production and release of IL-1). Many investigators use the comitogenic assay as a means of determining IL-1 activity in monocyte or macrophage supernatants. For large sample numbers microtiter methods are used.

## SELECTED REFERENCES

Allen, P. 1987. Antigen processing at the molecular level. *Immunol. Today.* 8(9):270.

Cohen, L., E. Pick, and J. Oppenheim, eds. 1979. *Biology of the lymphokines.* New York, NY: Academic Press.

Durum, S. K., J. A. Schmidt, and J. J. Oppenheim. 1985. Interleukin 1: An immunological perspective. *Ann. Rev. Immunol.* 3:263.

Gary, I., R. K. Gershon, and B. H. Waksman. 1972. Potentiation of the T lymphocyte response to mitogens. I. The responding cell. *J. Exp. Med.* 136:128.

Green, W. C., and W. C. Leonard. 1986. The human Interleukin-2 receptor. *Ann. Rev. Immunol.* 4:69.

Julius, M. H., E. Simpson, and L. A. Herzenberg. 1973. A rapid method for the isolation of functional thymus-derived murine lymphocytes. *Eur. J. Immunol.* 3:645.

Kaye, J., and C. A. Janeway, Jr., 1984. Induction of receptors for Interleukin-2 requires T cell Ag:Ia receptor crosslinking and Interleukin 1. *Lymphokine Res.* 3:175–182.

Marbrook, J. 1967. Primary immune response in cultures of spleen cells. *Lancet.* ii:1279.

Pierce, C. W., J. A. Kapp, and B. Benacerraf. 1976. Regulation by the H-2 gene complex of macrophage-lymphoid cell interactions in secondary antibody responses in vitro. *J. Exp. Med.* 144:371.

Robb, F. J. 1984. Interleukin 2. The molecule and its function. *Immunol. Today.* 5:203.

Schwartz, R. H. 1985. T-lymphocyte recognition of antigen in association with gene products of the major histocompatibility complex. *Ann. Rev. Immunol.* 3:237.

Unanue, E. R., and P. M. Allen. 1987. The basis for the immunoregulatory role of macrophages and other accessory cells. *Science.* 236:551.

# Selected Techniques

It would be a difficult task indeed to include in a single volume all the methods available (and important) to the contemporary immunologist. Many are simply too cumbersome; others require specialized equipment and instrumentation. Some require a time frame unsuitable for a laboratory period. Finally, many of them are expensive. However, a select group of procedures is not too time-consuming or too expensive, and rank so highly in importance to immunology that they should be included in a laboratory manual. This group has been selected for section V. The students' previous experiences should enable them to complete most of these exercises successfully.

**Column chromatographic procedures** have widespread use in cell biology and especially in immunology as indicated in exercise 12. However, one additional chromatographic method has been selected to provide the student with an in-depth experience in the preparation and use of columns. It involves the separation of components in a dialyzed serum sample. The serum is chromatographed on Sephadex G-200, and a fraction suspected of containing antibodies is collected and assayed for antibodies by double diffusion in agar. This exercise stresses the use of instrumentation in immunology and suggests the use of an integrated system of detection, recording, and collection devices.

**Immunoelectrophoresis** extends a previous exercise, and human serum is electrophoresed. Concepts of electrophoresis and gel diffusion are reviewed, and the result is related to clinical diagnosis of disease.

The **hemolytic plaque assay** holds great importance as the classic method to determine immune competence. As written, it allows the student to detect the ability of an animal to produce antibody to sheep red blood cells. The activity of complement as an immune response amplifier is stressed.

A **hypersensitivity** exercise is included because of the importance of pathological effects associated with some immune phenomena. It presents both B cell and T cell examples, but transplant immunology is a key component of this exercise. Students will transplant skin from one murine strain to another and follow the rejection process.

Finally, it presents an experiment that proves unequivocally that populations of **lymphocytes cooperate** to mount a successful immune response. It takes advantage of the fact that an irradiated mouse has an ablated immune system, and the mouse can be used in immune system reconstitution studies. Normal spleen cells and thymus cells or a combination of these are injected into irradiated mice, and the ability of the mice to respond to injected sheep red blood cells is determined. The hemolytic plaque assay studied previously indicates cell cooperation.

Taken together, the series of exercises from section V complements the student's growing list of accomplishments in the laboratory. Satisfactory results for each exercise depend on techniques developed in earlier procedures. Upon completion of these exercises, the student will have developed an extraordinary ability to **plan an experimental strategy, design the experiments** and **complete the experimentation.** Additionally, skills in **collection of data** and **interpretation of the results** will have been acquired.

*Figure V presents the approximate instructor preparation time and student laboratory time necessary for successful completion of Exercises 20 through 24.*

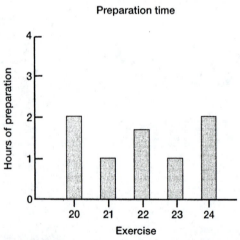

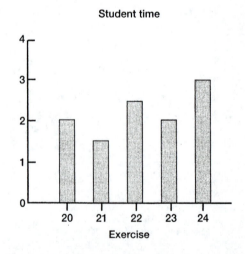

**FIGURE V**
Time allocation for Section V exercises.

# 20

# *Column Chromatography*

## INTRODUCTION

Proteins (including immunoglobulins) can be separated or fractionated by a number of different techniques collectively called **chromatography. Column chromatography** generally involves passing a protein mixture through a column containing a matrix of materials that retards the movement of specific proteins. In column chromatography each of the various proteins is retained differently depending on its interaction with the material in the column. The column itself is usually a glass or plastic tube, and the material chosen to be used in the chromatographic procedure is packed into it. Proteins that pass through are not chemically altered but separate on the basis of differences in charge, size or binding capacity.

Some materials (resins) used to prepare the matrix of the column may carry either a positive or negative charge. Proteins also carry a charge, and as they pass through the column, they attach to the charged resins. Proteins may be eluted sequentially as charges on the matrix are altered by changing the pH or molarity with eluting solution. This procedure is called **ion-exchange chromatography.** Diethylaminoethylcellulose (DEAE-cellulose) with a positive charge and carboxymethylcellulose (CM-cellulose) with a negative charge are insoluble matrix materials frequently used.

**Gel filtration** columns are packed with inert, porous beads. As protein solutions pass through the column, the small proteins (or other small molecules) enter the pores and are momentarily retained. They may pass through other beads as they continue down the column and again be retained. Eventually the larger, more rapidly moving molecules emerge from the column. The smaller molecules follow with continued elution. Various pore sizes facilitate separation of a variety of substances. The gel filtration method accurately determines the size and molecular weight of proteins. Popular gel filtration products are Sephadex, Sephacryl and Sepharose. Figure 20.1 shows the results of gel filtration using Sepharose to separate components of a mixture.

Finally, a specific protein can be separated from others by taking advantage of binding activities of proteins. The method, called **affinity chromatography,** was the subject of exercise 12 where it was used to purify a specific anti-

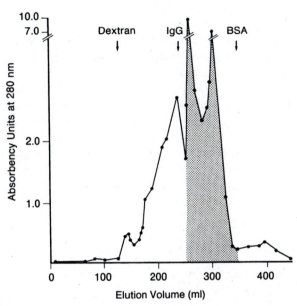

**FIGURE 20.1**

An example of the results obtained with gel filtration separation of a complex mixture. High-molecular-weight plasma components were fractionated on Sepharose CL in an attempt to determine the nature of the plasma cofactor that supports platelet aggregation of *Streptococcus salivarius.* It was demonstrated that fractions recovered in the shaded region (67,000 to 130,000 MW) supported platelet aggregations. The molecular weight standards used in this experiment were Dextran (2,000,000 MW), IgG and BSA.
Source: Sullam, Paul, M. *Infection and Immunity* 55 (1987);1747, figure 6.

body. For the purification, an **immunoadsorbant** is prepared by covalently coupling an antigen to an inert material such as agarose that is packed in a column. The mixture containing antibodies is added to the column; as the mixture travels down the matrix, the antibodies react with the immobilized antigen and are retained in the column. The antibodies can then be selectively eluted. One pass of a mixture through an affinity column can achieve significant purifications of proteins (up to 10,000-fold).

The sample to be column chromatographed in this exercise is a dialyzed rabbit serum sample. IgM, a specific component of rabbit serum, will be isolated in an effort to illustrate gel filtration methods. The process will exploit other important techniques such as dialysis.

The dialysis method permits a sample, such as serum containing low molecular weight materials, to be separated from these materials. If the serum is put in a semipermeable, membrane bag and placed in distilled water, the low molecular weight materials will diffuse through the membrane to equilibrate the concentration on both sides of the membrane. After several hours of dialysis, large molecules like IgM are retained and thus purified.

This exercise demonstrates principles of column chromatography beyond those learned in exercise 12. Although the exercise focuses on gel filtration chromatography of a serum sample, the student will also learn the preparation of column material, packing of the column, and use of auxiliary equipment. Specifically, a Sephadex G-200 column will be prepared and rabbit serum fractionated. Fractions will elute sequentially and eluted material will be monitored with a spectrophotometer at $A_{280}$. It is anticipated that IgM will elute early. Why? Fractions of eluent will be collected. An Ouchterlony double-diffusion test will be used to detect the presence of IgM and other rabbit serum proteins.

## MATERIALS

(Per pair)

Sephadex G-200 (Pharmacia, Inc., Piscataway, NJ)

Saline (0.85% NaCl)

Vacuum pump

Glass or plastic column (1 × 20 cm)

Buffer reservoir

Glassware

Dialysis tubing

Phosphate buffered saline (PBS) (pH 5.3) (See the appendix for the formulation)

Ultraviolet absorption monitor (spectrophotometer)

Fraction collector

Blue Dextran (Pharmacia, Inc., Piscataway, NJ)

Capillary pipettes

Rabbit serum (Serum from a rabbit injected 3 days previously with a heat-killed *Salmonella* species, or a commercially prepared sample)

Refrigerated centrifuge

Centrifuge tubes

1- and 5-ml pipettes

Distilled water

Ouchterlony double-diffusion agar in Petri dishes

Anti-rabbit serum

13 × 100-mm tubes

## PROCEDURE

1. Begin the preparation of the serum sample at least 3 days before needed. Collect 25 ml of **immune rabbit serum** (as described in exercise 1) and centrifuge in a high-speed refrigerated centrifuge (5,000 × g for 30 min) to remove aggregated lipids and other insoluble materials.

2. Pipette the clarified serum into tubular cellulose **dialysis tubing.** Some investigators prefer to soak the tubing overnight in water before using. Tie two knots in one end or use a dialysis clip before adding serum; after the addition of serum, tie two knots in the other end (or clip). Leave room to expand the tubing. If possible, do all of this work in the cold.

3. Dialysis occurs best if the loaded dialysis tubing is gently rotated or agitated in some way to enhance the movement of lower molecular weight molecules and salt ions. To do this, one could simply use a large reservoir containing distilled water and a stirring bar placed over a magnetic stirrer. The dialysis tubing may be free-floating in the liquid or suspended with string.

4. Change the distilled water in the reservoir every 6 to 8 hr for a 3-day period.

5. When the dialysis procedure is complete, protein will be precipitated. Open the dialysis tubing and transfer the contents to a centrifuge tube. Pellet the precipitate by centrifuging at 1,500 × g for 30 min in the cold.

6. Remove the supernatant and dissolve the pellet of precipitate in 5 ml of phosphate-buffered saline (PBS). Ideally, the precipitate in PBS should be stored overnight at 4° C to help the entire precipitate go back into solution.

7. Sephadex G-200 has a useful fractionation range of molecules with molecular weights of from 5,000 to 600,000 and will be used in this exercise to separate IgM from smaller immunoglobulins and other serum proteins. The Sephadex hydration procedure involves soaking Sephadex beads in saline for 3 days prior to use. Your instructor has added 1 g of Sephadex G-200 to 300 ml of saline and allowed it to soak for 3 days prior to class. It is important that there be no dissolved gasses in the saline used to prepare the column or in the eluting fluid. Dissolved gasses cause bubbles to form in the column once it has been prepared, and the imperfections that result will detain fractions. Prevent this by applying a vacuum to the Sephadex slurry for 1 hr prior to using. Prepare the eluting fluid the

same way. Be sure to discuss the details of column preparation with your instructor.

8. Choose a column that is approximately 20 cm in length and 1 cm wide. The bed volume should be approximately 35 ml/g of dry Sephadex. Mount the column **exactly vertical** on a ringstand with a means for adding eluting PBS. This can simply be a reservoir of eluting fluid mounted above the column and attached to it with tubing for gravity feed. Alternatively, use an automated fluid delivery system. Some columns keep the slurry from running out of the bottom of the column during preparation, but if not, plug the bottom of the column with glass wool. Provide a means at the bottom of the column for adjusting the flow rate of eluent out of the column. The **flow rate** of eluting fluid is critical.

9. Prepare the column by carefully pouring the Sephadex G-200 slurry into the column. Allow the Sephadex beads to settle. At the same time, allow the saline in the slurry to flow through and out of the column, but do not let the saline level fall below the top of the forming column. Continue to add slurry and continue to remove saline until a column of at least 18 cm high has been prepared. Be sure that the top of the column matrix is level and remains undisturbed.

10. Connect the eluting fluid reservoir to the column. Allow the eluting fluid, PBS (pH 5.3), to pass through the column for 15 min.

11. Students can monitor with spectroscopy the flow of **light-absorbing materials** out of the column. For this exercise the presence of protein in the eluting fluid shows up best with an ultraviolet adsorption monitor which takes a continuous reading of the effluent at $A_{280}$. Alternatively, students can collect fractions and take manual readings. Readings may be plotted continuously and samples collected according to volume with an automatic fraction collector (optional). Figure 20.2 shows an integrated system of instrumentation designed to: (1) monitor eluent for protein, and (2) collect samples of predetermined volume.

12. Before adding a serum sample to the column, determine the homogeneity of the bed by running a sample of Blue Dextran (2,000,000 MW) as described below. With this it is possible to determine how well the column was prepared by watching the progress of Blue Dextran as it moves down the column.

13. To load the column, elute the buffer to within 2 mm of the top of the Sephadex gel. Slowly add 1.0 ml of a 0.1% solution of Blue Dextran (in buffer) to the top of the gel with a capillary pipette. Be careful. **Do not disturb** the top of the column.

14. Open the column and allow buffer to elute dropwise. As this happens the Blue Dextran will enter the column. It is clearly visible because of the blue color. Close the column to keep the level of liquid at least 2 mm above the top of the column. Remember, do not let the liquid level fall below the top of the Sephadex bed.

15. Add additional buffer to the column and let it flow slowly into the gel bed. Finally, fill the column with buffer and attach to the buffer reservoir.

16. Set the flow rate to about 10 ml per hr. Collect the amount of eluting buffer necessary to move the Blue Dextran out of the column. The volume that elutes Blue Dextran is the **void volume.** Assume that IgM in the serum sample (to be added next) will pass through the column at about the time the void volume is eluted.

17. When the precipitate from step 6 has been redissolved, apply it to the Sephadex G-200 column as described for Blue Dextran. Collect the first protein fraction to come off the column. Do not dilute the sample during collection any more than necessary.

18. If done properly, the Sephadex G-200 should separate IgM from other proteins that co-precipitated in the dialysis tubing. Use the Ouchterlony double-diffusion method described in exercise 10 for testing the purity of the eluted protein.

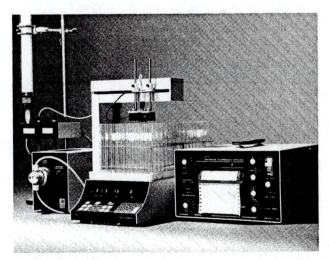

**FIGURE 20.2**
An integrated system for separation, identification, and collection of proteins. The column (left) separates components that flow through an absorbance monitor (below column) and are collected as fractions by a fraction collector (center). Readings are continuously monitored and recorded by an absorbance detector (right).
Courtesy of Isco, Inc.

19. Prepare double-diffusion plates with agar. Punch one center well and only two peripheral wells equal distance from the center well (about 6 mm).
20. Pipette anti-rabbit serum into the center well. Use precautions outlined earlier. Pipette the purified IgM from step 17 above into one of the peripheral wells. Pipette whole rabbit serum into the other well.
21. Incubate 24 to 48 hr and read the results. The double-diffusion technique should give you an indication of the purity of the IgM preparation. Explain.

## DISCUSSION

You may want to soak the dialysis tubing with several changes of distilled water to remove toxic materials. Alternatively, boil the tubing in distilled water.

In addition to the method described in this exercise, a number of other ways can remove proteins from serum. One popular method, **ammonium sulfate precipitation** (salting out) with subsequent dialysis or Sephadex G-25 desalting, is useful when attempting to purify IgG for DEAE chromatography. In addition, the Immersible-CX Ultrafilter (Millipore, Bedford, MA) or Centricon microconcentrators (Amicon, Beverly, MA) serve as excellent methods for concentrating protein.

The rabbit serum prepared for this exercise gives much better results if taken from an immune rabbit. A single injection of a bacterial species will give a high initial titer of IgM. An alternative to this exercise involves separating isoantibodies from human serum and detecting them with an agglutination procedure.

## SELECTED REFERENCES

Himmelhoch, S. R. 1971. Chromatography of proteins on ion-exchange adsorbents. *Meth. Enzymol.* 22:273.

Laurent, T. C., and J. Killander. 1964. A theory of gel filtration and its experimental verification. *K. Chromatogram* 14:317.

# 21

# *Immunoelectrophoresis*

## INTRODUCTION

Immunoelectrophoresis (IEP) serves as a powerful tool for the separation and detection of individual antigens present in a complex mixture. It goes a step further than electrophoresis by combining **electrophoresis** with **double gel diffusion.** The technique, first developed by Williams and Grabar, was reported in 1955.

In addition to accurately evaluating the presence and relative concentration of proteins in samples (serum or urine), immunoelectrophoresis can be used to determine if the proteins in the sample have been altered. This occurs in certain diseases like the monoclonal gammopathies.

When electrophoresis is used alone, the components of serum that have identical electrophoretic properties are not distinguishable from each other. IEP, however, further separates these components by their differences in diffusion rates in agar, followed by precipitation with antibody. Thus, individual components in a multi-component system can be identified, because the end result appears as precipitation of antigen and antibody in the agar matrix. Precipitation resulting from each antigen-antibody system produces an individual **arc of precipitation** (figure 21.1).

A high-purity agar should be used to eliminate nonspecific results. It is poured while hot onto clean microscope slides and allowed to harden on a level surface. (Prepared slides are also available commercially.) A special tool produces patterns of wells and troughs in the agar; the pattern chosen depends upon the application desired. The wells are carefully filled with the protein mixture to be separated, and the slides are placed in an electrophoretic chamber.

The pH of the buffer in the chamber is critical for maximum enhancement of protein movement. The application of a current for a predetermined time causes the components to separate. Safety is important when working with high voltage DC current (exercise 13). After electrophoresis, the trough, which is only a few millimeters away from the separated protein components, is filled with antiserum containing antibodies to proteins in the original sample. Upon incubation, both antigens and antibodies diffuse, and where they meet at equivalence, form an arc (figure 21.2). The mechanism of diffusion of antigen and antibody and subsequent reaction in agar resembles that seen in the Ouchterlony method (exercise 10).

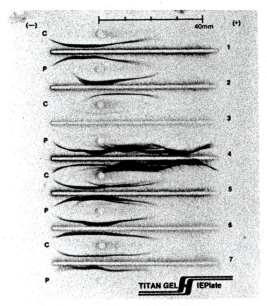

**FIGURE 21.1**

The results of immunoelectrophoresis of a patient's serum. The results indicate IgG lambda and IgA kappa monoclonal gammopathies. Notice the differences in the precipitation arcs of control and patient serum. The differences indicate protein structural abnormalities.
1 = IgG, 2 = IgA, 3 = IgM, 4 = Polyvalent, 5 = Trivalent, 6 = Kappa, 7 = Lambda antisera. C = Control and P = Patient.
Courtesy of Helena Laboratories

## MATERIALS

(Per pair)

       Immunoelectrophoretic agar (1% purified agar)

       Barbital buffer (pH 8.6)

       Ethyl alcohol (70%)

       Microscope slides

       Adhesive agar (0.1%) with glycerol (0.05%)

       Level

       5-ml pipette

       Agar cutter

       Human serum

       Tuberculin syringe with 23-gauge needle

       Electrophoresis apparatus

       Filter paper strips

       Anti-human serum

       Moist chamber

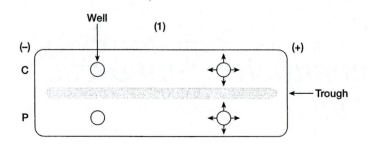

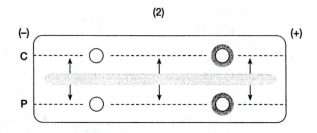

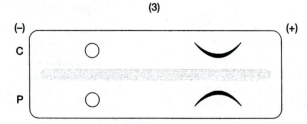

**FIGURE 21.2**
The mechanism of immunoelectrophoresis. (1) After electrophoresis of protein (e.g., patient's serum), the separated components begin to diffuse radially (only one component is shown here for descriptive purposes). (2) Antiserum is added to the trough after electrophoresis, and diffuses into the agar in the direction of the arrows. (3) When antigen and antiserum meet at equivalence in the agar, precipitation results forming an arc. If arcs produced by antigen in patient's serum are abnormal as compared to controls, a specific disease is indicated. C = Control and P = Patient.

## PROCEDURE

1. Prepare immunoelectrophoretic agar in barbital buffer (pH 8.6; see the appendix for the formulation of barbital buffer) with 1% purified agar. Melt and hold the agar at 60° C.

2. Use ethyl alcohol-cleaned microscope slides. After cleaning, dip each slide into a mixture of melted adhesive agar containing glycerol (0.1% agar, 0.05% glycerol plus water). Slant and allow the slides to dry. This step assures that the immunoelectrophoretic agar will attach firmly when poured on the slide and keeps the sample from running under the immunoelectrophoretic agar.

3. To minimize differences in agar thickness over the length of the slide, position the slide so that it is exactly level. Pipette 2 ml of melted immunoelectrophoretic agar onto the slide (use a prewarmed pipette). Add the agar slowly and do not allow it to run off the edge of the slide. The agar should harden quickly and have a **uniform depth** of a few millimeters. Allow the agar to solidify at room temperature.

4. Use an immunoelectrophoresis agar cutter especially designed to cut specific electrophoretic patterns. The cutters available from a number of vendors fit over the slide and punch a predetermined pattern. Punch the wells. A commonly used pattern appears in figure 21.1. Carefully suction out the agar plug from the cut wells. Avoid ragged edges.

5. Carefully fill the wells with human serum. Use a tuberculin syringe fitted with a 23-gauge needle. Do not overfill.

6. Fill the reservoirs of an electrophoresis chamber with barbital buffer (pH 8.6). Position the slide in the chamber. Follow your instructor's directions. Make contact between the agar on each end of the slide and the buffer in the reservoirs with filter paper strips that have been saturated with buffer. Each strip should touch the agar only at the very end of the slide and dip into the buffer in the reservoir.

7. Connect the power supply and turn it on. Slowly increase the voltage to approximately 150 volts. This should provide a 2 milliampere current through the agar. When the current is on, it will move from one electrode in one chamber through the buffer, through one filter paper strip, through the agar on the slide, through the other filter paper strip into buffer in the other reservoir, and finally to the other electrode. When the circuit is complete, the charged components in the sample will begin to move.

8. Allow electrophoresis to continue for 60 min and turn off the power. Remove the slide from the chamber.

9. Since the pattern cut earlier included the trough, simply remove the agar with a sharp blade to produce the trough. Carefully add anti-human serum to the trough with a tuberculin syringe with a 23-gauge needle.

10. Place the slide in a moist chamber at room temperature.

11. Read the precipitation arcs that develop within 24 to 48 hr.

## DISCUSSION

This procedure can be altered depending upon the results desired. For example, either antigens or antibodies can be electrophoresed. In the clinical laboratory it may be desirable to detect human antibodies in serum. These antibodies would therefore serve as antigens and anti-human serum antibodies would be used to detect them.

Students should pay particular attention to the voltage and milliamperage. Most electrophoretic chambers accommodate several slides, and as the number increases, the current will have to be adjusted accordingly. Why?

The precipitation arcs produced by IEP appear without staining, but one may wish to stain with a protein stain such as acid fuchsin to make the arcs more visible. Several other stains are also available, and the choice depends upon the usefulness of a particular stain to the investigator. After staining, sequential washes removes excess stain. As many as 20 different antigenic components in human serum may be resolved; this makes the technique useful in clinical diagnosis of disease. Most of the time, normal and abnormal sera are assayed on the same slide for comparison purposes. This makes it easy to recognize anomalies. Additionally, the IEP method has many research applications.

The arcs should be clear, precise and three-dimensional. **Excess precipitate** can result from serum overload and may require dilution of serum or antibody. Unusual results, however, may indicate above-normal serum protein levels. This is the case when the precipitation arcs are thicker and closer to the trough than normal. This makes the method semiquantitative.

## SELECTED REFERENCES

Caron, J., and G. M. Penn 1992. Electrophoretic and immunochemical characterization of immunoglobulins. In *Manual of clinical laboratory immunology.* 4th ed. Edited by N. R. Rose, E. C. de Macario, J. L. Fahely, H. Friedman, and G. M. Penn. Washington, DC: American Society for Microbiology.

Weir, D. M., L. A. Herzenberg, C. Blackwell, Leonore A. Herzenberg, eds. 1986. Handbook of experimental immunology. 4th ed. Oxford: Blackwell Scientific Publications.

Williams, C. A., Jr., and P. Grabar. 1955. Immunoelectrophoretic studies of serum proteins. I. The antigens of human serum. *J. Immunol.* 74:158.

Williams, C. A., Jr., and P. Grabar. 1955. Immunoelectrophoretic studies of serum proteins. II. Immune sera: antibody distribution. *J. Immunol.* 74:397.

# *Hemolytic Plaque Assay*

## INTRODUCTION

This exercise detects lymphocytes that are producing high-efficiency, lysing antibodies. The described procedure allows the identification of a **single lymphocyte** that is producing specific antibody from within a large population of cells. The basic technique indicates only those cells secreting IgM antibody.

IgM fixes complement with great efficiency, a necessity for antibodies designed to lyse target cells. A single molecule of IgM attached to a sheep red blood cell (SRBC) is sufficient to initiate lysis of the target SRBC, but the complement cascade finally brings about lysis.

Jerne and Nordin developed the assay in 1963, but since then a number of modifications have been reported, including both **direct** and **indirect methods** and also methods that provide fluorescent staining of results. Others combine autoradiographic techniques with the plaque assay. Modifications depend upon the application of the technique. Figure 22.1 describes the classical results of Mitchell and Miller that laid the groundwork for our understanding of **T and B cell function.** The hemolytic plaque assay provided the means for them to answer questions concerning basic fundamentals of immunology. Rather than directly measure the amount of antibody produced, they chose to count spleen cells that secrete antibody specific for SRBC.

The **direct method** serves as the most useful method for the immunology student. Mice are immunized with a large inoculate of SRBC to elicit a primary antibody response. Lymphocytes become sensitized to the large number of antigenic determinants on the SRBC, antibody production begins, and the titer of IgM antibodies rises over a period of about four days. The immune mouse is killed, the spleen is removed, and a single-cell suspension of spleen cells is made. These are mixed with a dense suspension of SRBC. This mixture is incorporated into an agar support medium and poured in a thin layer in a Petri dish. All cells are thereby essentially immobilized within the agar.

During an incubation period, sensitized lymphocytes secrete antibody that diffuses through the agar and reacts with SRBC, the indicator cells. The complement cascade, initiated upon addition of complement, results in lysis of the SRBC. A clear area surrounding the antibody-producing cell is produced and is called a **plaque.** Results are usually expressed as plaques counted.

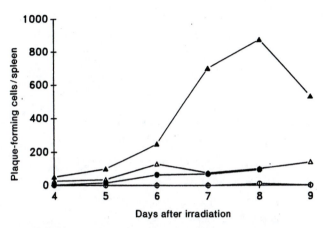

**FIGURE 22.1**

Plaque-forming cells produced in spleens of heavily irradiated mice whose immune systems have been reconstituted with immune cells or combinations of them and then injected with SRBC. (○), SRBC alone; (●), SRBC and syngeneic thoracic duct cells; (△), SRBC and syngeneic bone marrow cells; (▲), SRBC, syngeneic bone marrow and thoracic duct cells. These results indicate that the injection of bone marrow and thoracic duct cells in combination greatly increases the number of plaque-forming cells produced over the number produced by either of these cells alone.

From Miller and Mitchell, *Journal of Experimental Medicine*, 1968. Reproduced by copyright permission of The Rockefeller University Press.

This **quantitative** assay provides a determination of absolute numbers of antibody-producing cells. However, it is not useful for determining the concentration of antibodies.

Antibody-producing cells must secrete adequate antibody for lysis of a sufficient number of SRBC to produce visible plaques. High-affinity antibodies produce smaller plaques. Likewise, a high density of antigenic determinants on the SRBC also produces small plaques.

The direct method can be extended to measure the production of other classes of antibodies such as IgG (figure 22.2). IgG antibodies will attach to SRBC but fail to lyse them even in the presence of complement. An **anti-Ig serum** can be added that will attach to the IgG molecules already attached to the SRBC. Upon addition of complement, the anti-Ig antibodies will **facilitate the lysis** of the target cell by IgG. To determine the number of cells that form plaques by the **indirect method** (and thus the number of IgG-secreting cells), one can subtract the number of plaques detected by the indirect method from those detected by the direct method.

The basic plate method (direct) follows as originally described with a few modifications. It has advantages over other methods in that a larger number of plaques can be counted, thereby increasing the reliability of the method.

## MATERIALS

(Per pair)

HEPES-buffered balanced salt solution (HEPES-BSS)

1 mouse immunized IP 4 days before needed with a 5% suspension of SRBC (experimental)

1 mouse not immunized (control)

6 plates of 1.5% purified agar in HEPES-BSS

6 tubes of top agar (0.7% purified agar in HEPES-BSS plus 1 mg/ml DEAE-dextran)

1 tube 15% washed SRBC in HEPES-BSS

1 tube guinea pig complement (diluted 1:10)

Surgical instruments

Ice bath

Sterile Petri dishes (15 × 60 mm)

Sterile capillary pipettes

Sterile 13 × 100-mm tubes

Unopette® white cell pipette

WBC diluting fluid

Hemacytometer with coverslips

Counters

Pipettes (0.5-, 1.0- and 5.0-ml)

Tuberculin needle and syringe

Purified agar

37° C incubator and water bath

45° C water bath

DEAE-dextran (Pharmacia, Inc., Piscataway, NJ)

Sterile rubber policeman

Centrifuge

Moist chamber

$CO_2$ for mouse euthanasia

Tubes for dilution series

## PROCEDURE

1.  Immunize mice intraperitoneally 4 days before needed with 1 ml of a 5% washed SRBC suspension.
2.  Prepare 1.5% purified agar in HEPES-buffered balanced salt solution (HEPES-BSS). The formulation for the balanced salt solution is presented in the appendix. Pour 6 ml into each of six, 15 × 60-mm Petri dishes. Prepare these 2 or

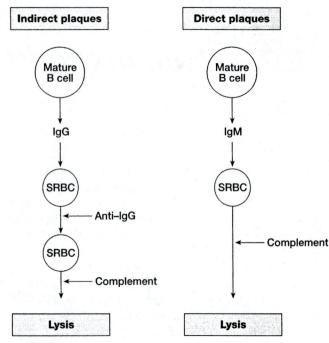

**FIGURE 22.2**
The mechanisms for producing indirect or direct plaques. Plaques result from lysis of target cells by antibody.

3 days prior to use and store at 4° C in a moist chamber. Warm to 37° C before use. This agar will provide a base for the top agar added later.

3.  Prepare a top agar by mixing 0.7% purified agar with HEPES-BSS. Add 1 mg/ml DEAE-dextran to remove anticomplementary factors present in the agar. Heat to dissolve the agar and DEAE-dextran.

4.  Place 6 small tubes in a rack and put in a 45° C water bath. Pipette 2 ml of hot top agar into each.

5.  Wash SRBC 3 times in HEPES-BSS (centrifuge at 250 × g for 10 min each wash) and resuspend to a 15% suspension in HEPES-BSS. Hold at 37° C until needed.

6.  Dilute guinea pig complement 1:10 in HEPES-BSS and prewarm to 37° C in a water bath. Hold until needed.

7.  Kill the **immunized and control mice** with $CO_2$ as outlined in exercise 4. Aseptically remove the spleens as discussed in exercise 11 and place them in sterile Petri dishes. Properly label the dishes with **control** for the nonimmunized mouse and **experimental** for the immunized mouse. It is good practice to follow aseptic procedure even though microbial contamination may have no adverse effect on the results of this exercise.

8. Add 5 ml of prewarmed HEPES-BSS to each culture dish and carefully open each spleen with a sharp scalpel. Tease the spleen apart with a sterile rubber policeman as previously described and attempt to produce a suspension of **individual spleen cells.** Do not leave clumps of spleen. Some prefer to force fragments of the spleen through a small wire mesh to produce a single-cell suspension.

9. Remove the cells with a sterile capillary pipette, place in a centrifuge tube, and spin at 250 × g for 5 min.

10. Discard the supernatant and wash the cells with 5 ml of cold HEPES-BSS. Centrifuge at 250 × g for 5 min.

11. Resuspend the cell pellet in 1 ml of cold HEPES-BSS. Hold the cells in an ice bath while determining the cell count.

12. Do this by preparing a 1:20 dilution using a Unopette® white cell pipette and white blood cell diluting fluid. This procedure was described in exercise 3. Add to a hemacytometer and determine the number of cells in the suspension.

13. Dilute the cell suspension to $2.5 \times 10^7$ cells/ml with HEPES-BSS.

14. Carefully pipette 0.2 ml of the **SRBC suspension** from step 5 into each of the 6 tubes of top agar which have been tempered to 45° C in a water bath (step 4).

15. Use a 0.5-ml and 1.0-ml pipette to add 0.05, 0.2, 0.3, 0.4, 0.5, and 0.6 ml of the **spleen cell suspension** to the individual tubes of top agar. This dilution procedure should give a countable plate.

16. Rapidly, but gently, mix and pour each tube of top agar plus cells over the surface of a plate prepared in step 2. Be careful not to allow the soft top agar to solidify in the tube or during pouring, because artifacts may be produced. Tilt the plate to obtain a smooth and even top agar. Allow to solidify.

17. Incubate the plates for 1 hr at 37° C in a humidified incubator.

18. After the 1 hr incubation period is complete, add 2 ml of diluted complement prepared in step 6 to each of the plates. Slowly rotate the plate to spread the complement over the entire surface. Be careful not to tear the top agar layer.

19. Incubate once again at 37° C for 0.5 to 1 hr.

20. Observe the plaques.

## DISCUSSION

Plaques are best seen with the aid of a dissecting microscope. They appear as small, round, clear areas against a red cell background. With higher magnifications, one can observe a **lymphocyte at the center** of the plaque. If desired, complement can be poured off, and the red cells stained with benzidine dihydrochloride or O-tolidine for better resolution of the plaques. When benzidine is used, the red cell background stains dark blue.

Of course, there can be too few or too many plaques per plate. A good number is between 100 and 200. The dilution procedure in step 15 provides a plate with the appropriate number of plaques for counting. The results may be expressed as **plaque forming cells (PFC)** per spleen or per number of spleen cells added.

## SELECTED REFERENCES

Jerne, N. K., C. Henry, A. A. Nordin, H. Fuji, A.M.C. Koros, and I. Lefkovits. 1974. Plaque-forming cells: Methodology and theory. *Transplant. Rev.* 18:130.

Jerne, N. K., and A. A. Nordin. 1963. Plaque formation by single antibody-producing cells. *Science.* 140:405.

Mitchell, G. F., and J. F. A. P. Miller 1968. Cell-to-cell interaction in the immune response. II. The source of hemolysin-forming cells in irradiated mice given bone marrow and thymus or thoracic duct lymphocytes. *J. Exp. Med.* 128:821.

Plotz, P. H., N. Talal, and R. Asofsky. 1968. Assignment of direct and facilitated hemolytic plaques in mice to specific immunoglobulin classes. *J. Immunol.* 100:744.

Sell, S., A. B. Park, and A. A. Nordin. 1970. Immunoglobulin classes of antibody-forming cells in mice. I. Localized hemolysis-in-agar plaque-forming cells belonging to five immunoglobulin classes. *J. Immunol.* 104:483.

Serge, D., and M. Serge. 1976. Visualization of plaque-forming cells in agar plates stained with O-tolidine. *J. Immunol. Meth.* 12:197.

# 23

# *Hypersensitivity*

## INTRODUCTION

In contrast to the immune responses that protect against disease, some immune reactions lead to tissue damage. These detrimental phenomena, collectively known as **hypersensitivity,** result once the individual has been primed with particular antigens. The term **allergen** indicates the sensitizing material that causes the symptoms usually associated with a hyperimmune reaction. Some prefer to use the term **allergy,** a synonym for hypersensitivity.

The antibodies or sensitized cells that result are produced in relatively large numbers, and, when contact is made with specific antigen, the classic reactions of hypersensitivity result. Results of hypersensitivity may be: (1) anaphylaxis, (2) antibody-dependent cytotoxic hypersensitivity, (3) a complex-mediated reaction, or (4) a cell-mediated reaction.

The reaction may take place immediately—an **immediate reaction**—or it may be **delayed.** Immediate reactions take place within seconds to 4 to 6 hours after exposure, and the delayed reaction takes 24 to 48 hours. Antibodies are responsible for immediate reactions while sensitized cells are responsible for delayed reactions.

**Anaphylactic sensitivities** result when antibodies bind to mast cells (or basophils) by the Fc portion of the antibody molecule, and this combination encounters the antigen. As a consequence of the resulting antigen-antibody reaction, the mast cell degranulates, releasing a number of pharmacologic **vasoactive substances.** These substances incite some harmful responses such as dilation of blood vessels and contraction of smooth muscle (figure 23.1).

**Antibody-dependent cytotoxic hypersensitivities** result from antibodies produced to some of the cell surface antigens present on lymphoreticular cells (target cells). When these antibodies react with the target cell, complement is activated, and the target cell is killed by complement-dependent lysis. Immunoadherence reactions involving complement and phagocytic cells are also antibody-dependent and can lead to phagocytosis and death of target cells.

Often, antigen and antibody complexes lead to **acute inflammatory reactions.** Complement is activated, and this causes mast cell histamine release or polymorphonuclear cell release of proteolytic enzymes. The end result is amplification of the inflammatory response and damage to tissue. Figure 23.2 shows the events that occur.

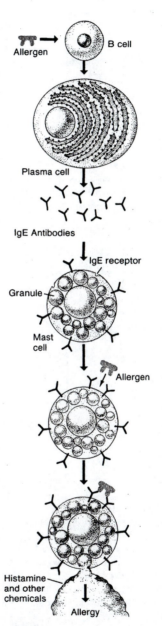

**FIGURE 23.1**
Allergy (anaphylactic sensitivity) results when antibodies of the IgE class produced by plasma cells attach to tissue mast cells. The combination of these antibodies with allergens (antigens that provoke an allergic reaction) cause the mast cell to secrete vasoactive substances, including histamine, that produce the symptoms of allergy.

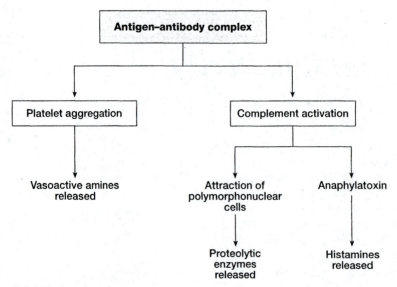

**FIGURE 23.2**
Antigen-antibody complex may initiate a series of hypersensitivity events that result in the production of mediators that can damage the host. The result is an acute inflammatory reaction.

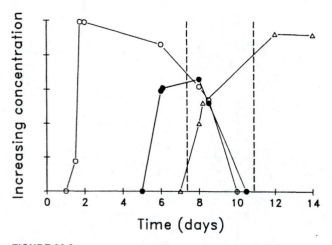

**FIGURE 23.3**
The in vivo events of serum sickness. An antigen is injected and is present in the serum for a period of several days. During that time, antibody production begins and antibodies react with remaining antigen. Complexes are formed that are deposited on vascular walls producing the symptoms of the disease. As antigen is removed from the circulation in the antigen-antibody complexes, free antibody titer begins to rise. The period of time represented on the graph by the dashed vertical lines represents the duration of disease. (○), circulating free antigen; (●), circulating antigen-antibody complexes; (△), circulating free antibody.

Another antigen-antibody complex-mediated hypersensitivity is **serum sickness.** After contact with antigen, individuals produce antibodies that react with the remaining circulating antigen. Complexes form and activate complement that, in turn, causes liberation of vasoactive substances. Antigen-antibody complexes may be deposited in the blood vessel walls and produce severe arteritis. Likewise, the complexes can localize in the glomeruli of the kidney and cause glomerulonephritis. Figure 23.3 graphically illustrates the events that occur during serum sickness.

**Cell-mediated hypersensitivity** results from stimulated and consequently sensitized T cells. In one example, the antigens on certain cells (such as transplanted tissue) are the targets of sensitized cells, and the reaction results in death of the antigen-bearing cell. Cell-mediated hypersensitivities may also involve the release of lymphokines.

The experiments presented in this exercise demonstrate some of these hypersensitivities. The first will be **anaphylactic shock.** A guinea pig will be sensitized to antigen, and, after a suitable time, the shocking dose of antigen will be administered. A typical anaphylactic reaction should result. The author recommends that this part of the exercise be done as a class experiment to avoid unnecessary use of experimental animals or, alternatively, show a video tape of the experiment.

The second experiment involves an antigen-antibody complex that produces a visible, localized tissue reaction, **passive cutaneous anaphylaxis.** A guinea pig will be injected intradermally with an antiserum and 4 to 6 hours later the homologous antigen and a dye will be injected intravenously. As a consequence of the antigen-antibody reaction that follows, histamine will be released, causing capillary permeability to increase. The damage at the site of the antiserum injection will appear within 15 minutes as indicated by dye that escapes from the vessels into surrounding tissue because of the damage.

An **allograft (homograft) rejection reaction** will demonstrate a cell-mediated hypersensitivity reaction. Skin grafts (mouse tail skin) will be placed on isogenic and allogenic recipients. The **isogenic recipient** is one that is genetically identical to the donor and the **allogenic recipient** is from the same species but genetically different from the donor. The isogenic recipients will serve as controls. Within a period of 7 to 14 days the allogenic graft will be rejected because of sensitization of recipient cells to surface antigens on donor cells.

## MATERIALS

(Per class and student pair)

    2 guinea pigs

    Horse serum

    Tuberculin syringes and needles

    21- and 27-gauge needles

    Surgical instruments (scissors, scalpel, forceps, hemostats)

    Ethanol (70%)

    Anti-BSA

    Sterile saline

    0.25% BSA and 2% Evans Blue mixture

    3-ml syringes

    Ketamine-xylazine anesthesia (see appendix)

    Nembutal (injectable sodium pentathal, a controlled substance)

    BALB/c mice (white)

    C57 mice (black)

    Animal clippers

    Surgical tape

    Betadine soap

    Sterile Petri dishes

    Phosphate buffered saline (PBS) (pH 7.2)

    Filter paper

    $CO_2$ for mouse euthanasia

    Silk sutures and needles (optional)

    Sterile gauze pads (Vaseline impregnated)

    Heat lamp

    Razor or single-edge razor blade

    Marking pen

    Small culture tubes

    Surgical table (optional)

    Balance for mouse weights

## PROCEDURE

## Anaphylactic Shock

(Class Experiment)

1. Three weeks prior to producing anaphylactic shock in a guinea pig, make intraperitoneal injections of 0.1 ml of horse serum or other appropriate soluble antigens intraperitoneally on three alternate days. Use the procedure described in exercise 1 for intraperitoneal injection.

2. To produce anaphylactic shock, inject the shocking dose of antigen (3 ml of horse serum) into the heart. Do not anesthetize the guinea pig. Have an assistant hold the animal on its back. Insert the needle containing horse serum, aspirate to make certain the needle is in the heart and inject quickly. For more specific information, use the procedure outlined in exercise 1 that describes bleeding from the heart.

3. Within a few minutes after administration of the shocking dose, the guinea pig will exhibit cardinal signs of **systemic anaphylactic shock.** The animal will begin to cough and gasp for air. It will paw at its nose and become convulsive. Death will result within 5 min.

4. Autopsy the guinea pig and note the condition of the lungs. What did you find?

## Passive Cutaneous Anaphylaxis (PCA)

(Class Experiment)

1. Remove the hair from the back of a white guinea pig with electric clippers and then shave the same area with a razor. A single-edge razor blade and soap works well. Wash the shaved area with 70% alcohol.

2. Use a black marking pen to circle 4 well-separated areas where intradermal injections will be made. Label appropriately.

3. Inject one area with 0.1 ml of sterile saline to serve as the control. Inject other areas with: (1) undiluted anti-BSA, (2) anti-BSA diluted 1:10 with saline, and (3) anti-BSA diluted 1:100 with saline. Use tuberculin syringes and needles. All injections should be intradermal by the following method. First wipe the area with 70% ethanol. Insert the needle slowly into the skin at a 20-degree angle with the bevel of the needle up. Once in the skin, continue to insert the needle but do this parallel to the skin. Stop when about 2 mm of the needle is in the skin. Inject slowly.

The injection will produce a bleb (a raised, blanched area) if done properly. Withdraw the needle and wipe the area with 70% ethanol.

4. Allow the animal to rest for 4 to 6 hr.

5. In the meantime prepare a mixture of BSA and Evans Blue dye. Use equal volumes of 0.25% BSA and 2% Evans Blue.

6. Inject 1 ml of the BSA-Evans Blue solution intravenously. Do this via the marginal ear vein or, if the guinea pig is small and intravenous injection into the marginal ear vein is difficult, try the saphenous vein in the leg or make the injection into the heart.

7. Observe the labelled areas where antiserum was injected for 15 to 45 min after injection of the BSA-Evans Blue solution.

8. A reaction is positive when the skin at the antiserum injection sites turns blue. A maximum reaction may be seen within 15 min. Compare to the control site.

## Allograft Rejection

(Pairs of Students)

1. Use two different strains of inbred mice. A **black C57** mouse will serve as the tissue donor and a **white BALB/c** mouse will serve as the recipient. Each pair of students will use two donors and two recipients. Skin from the tail will be transplanted from the C57 mouse to the thorax area of a BALB/c mouse. As a control, tail skin will be removed from another BALB/c mouse and attached to the thoracic area of another BALB/c mouse as outlined below. To emphasize the recognition of self-antigens, reverse the skin on the control so that the hair grows in the reverse direction.

2. This surgical transplantation procedure requires the recipient animal to be anesthetized with ketamine-xylazine anesthesia (see appendix) or with Nembutal (0.06 mg/g of mouse body weight) injected intraperitoneally. The donors should be killed in $CO_2$. It also requires strict adherence to directions presented by the instructor for proper removal of skin and transplantation onto a recipient. Strict aseptic technique is not required, but use care in the procedure to prevent infection. For example, keep surgical instruments in a 70% ethanol beaker and simply wipe on gauze before use.

3. The student should plan the timing of each step carefully. Kill a C57 and BALB/c mouse when ready to prepare the transplant skin and be prepared to anesthetize the two BALB/c mice

when the transplant skin is ready. (Note: A single mouse of each strain may provide enough tail skin for several student pairs, which will prevent excessive use of donor mice.)

4. At this point, prepare the mice for skin transplantation using the following procedures:

   a. To prepare tail skin from the donor, swab the tail of the dead C57 mouse with 70% ethanol or a disinfectant soap such as Betadine. Make a longitudinal cut from the base of the tail down the dorsal surface. Make a circumferential cut at the base of the tail and another at the end of the longitudinal cut. Grasp the skin with forceps and peel away from the cartilaginous tail. Place the skin into a sterile Petri dish. A piece of filter paper placed in the dish and moistened with PBS (pH 7.2) will keep the skin moist during the next step.

   b. To prepare the site to attach transplanted tail skin, anesthetize the mouse and secure the mice to a surgical table (or some other table top) that has been disinfected. Follow the instructor's directions. Leave the graft area exposed. Remove the hair from the thorax and abdominal areas of the BALB/c mice with animal clippers. Shave the area on the right side of the thorax (over the ribs) with a razor or a single-edge razor blade and soap. Wash the skin with 70% ethanol.

5. Using forceps and dissecting scissors, trim the tail skin to produce a square (approximately 5 mm on each side). See figure 23.4 for a diagram of the skin. Place the tissue back into the Petri dish on the wet filter paper with the epidermis side up. The tail skin will remain viable for hours at room temperature.

6. Clean and sterilize the graft areas completely once again. Use 70% ethanol or a disinfectant soap such as Betadine.

7. After determining the exact area for the graft placement (approximately 4 mm square), pinch one side of the square of skin with small forceps. Using dissecting scissors, cut the skin as superficially as possible. The tissue directly beneath the dermis must remain intact so that blood and lymph vessels found there can sustain the transplanted tissue. The blood supply to the newly transplanted tissue will come from the vessels in the panniculus carnosus. This small, transparent muscle layer lies on top of the muscle tissue. It can be distinguished by the numerous blood vessels and by the fact that it can be moved around over the underlying muscle.

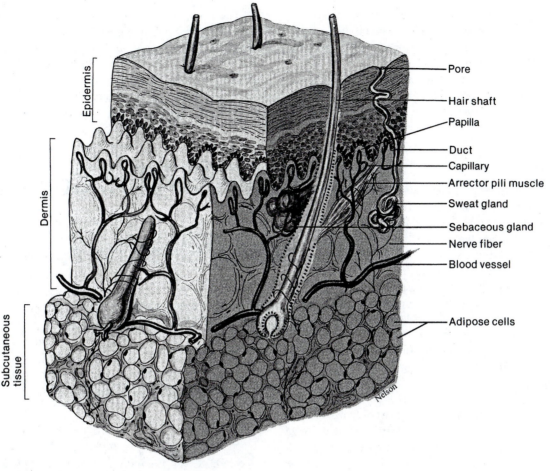

Epidermis

Dermis

Subcutaneous tissue

Pore

Hair shaft

Papilla

Duct

Capillary

Arrector pili muscle

Sweat gland

Sebaceous gland

Nerve fiber

Blood vessel

Adipose cells

Nelson

**FIGURE 23.4**
A diagram illustrating the structure of the skin.
From John W. Hole, Jr., *Human Anatomy and Physiology*, 3d ed. Copyright © 1984 Wm. C. Brown Publishers, Dubuque, Iowa. All Rights Reserved. Reprinted by permission.

8. Complete excision of the tissue by cutting along each of the 4 sides of the square. Then carefully pull the tissues away from the mouse by working from each of the 4 corners sequentially and pulling toward the center of the square. Finally lift off the skin. (Important: Do not damage the panniculus.) Discard the square of tissue.

9. The graft bed should be smaller in diameter (approximately 4 mm) than the donor tissue since the graft will shrink somewhat. Work quickly so that the graft bed does not dry out. Moisten the area periodically with sterile saline or PBS. If bleeding occurs, simply remove the blood with sterile gauze.

10. Place the C57 tail skin graft onto the graft bed. Carefully smooth out the wrinkles to assure a good fit.

11. At this point the graft may be: (1) sutured into place, or (2) held in place with a compress bandage. The instructor may demonstrate both methods.

12. To suture, use 5–0 silk sutures and place 4 to 8 sutures at appropriate sites around the grafted tissue. Then apply a surgical dressing.

13. Alternatively, carefully place a Vaseline-impregnated gauze on the graft. Hold this **tightly** in place with surgical tape or a plaster bandage.

14. Repeat the procedure with the **control mice.**

15. Place the animals in a warm place (under a heat lamp) until they recover from the anesthesia.

16. Cage the animals and observe periodically.

17. If bandages were applied, anesthetize the mouse and carefully remove the bandages after 7 days. When removing them be sure that the transplanted tissue did not stick to the gauze. Moisten the bandages with saline or buffer to prevent sticking. If rejection has already occurred, the graft may come off with the bandages anyway.

18. Observe the grafts. The grafted tissue on the control should appear rather pale but nevertheless adhere to the animal. The graft

should not have shrunk away from the margins of the bed and there should be no inflammation to suggest infection. Attachment at the margins of the graft should be obvious. The **allografts** should be well on their way toward **rejection.** They will be discolored and contracted with no attachment at the margins. Necrosis of the grafted tissue will be obvious.

## DISCUSSION

Anaphylaxis, an immediate, obvious, and impressive reaction, demonstrates the **disastrous effects** of some hypersensitivities. Very small amounts of antigen (e.g., bee venom) can sometimes initiate the reaction with effects exerted on vascular and smooth muscles. Results of anaphylaxis can be reversed by immediate administration of **epinephrine** which prevents degranulation of mast cells and, in addition, counteracts the effect of histamine on smooth muscle. Upon autopsy of the guinea pig, students should realize that the animal suffocated because of the inability to exhale. The lungs will appear extended. Students may also detect vascular damage by carefully looking at the lungs for small hemorrhages.

The passive cutaneous anaphylaxis experiment also provides visual evidence of the consequences of hypersensitivity reactions. The results are easily interpreted as **damage to tissue,** specifically an increase in vascular permeability allowing dye and serum to escape from blood vessels. The injected antigen reacts with injected antibody and triggers degranulation at the site of the injection.

The final experiment involving transplant rejection is easily interpreted as an immune phenomenon. The T cell is primarily responsible for the rejection of solid grafts, proven by showing that the **nude mouse** cannot reject skin grafts. Since MHC antigens on the allogeneic transplanted tissue are highly immunogenic, the response can be diminished in the recipient only by taking immunosuppressive measures.

## SELECTED REFERENCES

Askenase, P. W., and M. Van Loveren. 1983. Delayed-type hypersensitivity: Activation of mast cells by antigen-specific T-cell factors initiates the cascade of cellular interactions. *Immunol. Today.* 4:259.

Beal, G. N., ed. 1983. *Allergy and clinical immunology.* New York, NY: John Wiley and Sons.

Befus, A. K., J. Bienenstock, and J. A. Denburg. 1985. Mast cell differentiation and heterogenity. *Immunol. Today.* 6:281.

Ishizaka, K. 1984. Regulation of IgE synthesis. *Ann. Rev. Immunol.* 2:159.

Lockey, R. F., and S. C. Bukantz, eds. 1987. Principles of immunology and allergy. Philadelphia, PA: W. B. Saunders.

Naguwa, S. M., and B. L. Nelson. 1985. Human serum sickness. *Clin. Rev. Allergy.* 3:117.

Yoshida, T., ed. 1985. *Investigation of cell-mediated immunity.* Edinburg: Churchill Livingstone.

# 24

# *Cell Cooperation*

## INTRODUCTION

With all our knowledge of cell biology, many questions remain unanswered. One involves cellular communication. Immunologists strive to unravel the mysteries that surround the cellular communications that lead to an appropriate immune response. Claman, Chaperon and Triplett in 1966 first described the existence of cellular interactions between lymphocytes that are necessary to mount an immune response to sheep red blood cells (SRBC).

Specifically, they showed that the combination of adult **marrow and thymus cells** produce more anti-sheep red blood cell hemolysin than the sum of the separate cell populations. Adult thymus also acts with adult spleen cells to produce a significant response. This work began our understanding of the importance of combinations of cells for certain immune responses.

These experiments were possible at that time because of a knowledge of the effect of irradiation on mice. Mice exposed to 650–750 r of total body irradiation (ionizing radiation) become immunologically suppressed because of the effects produced on the biochemical and functional properties of lymphocytes. Lymphocytes are particularly radiosensitive, so their function can be totally abolished with x-irradiation. The radiation dosage necessary for immunosuppression is less than the $LD_{50}$ for mice, but death follows two weeks later because of failure of the hemopoietic system. Between irradiation and death, the mouse serves as a living test tube. Its immune system can be reconstituted by injecting various populations of syngeneic (genetically identical) cells. After reconstitution, the mouse can be challenged with antigen and the response (or lack of response) measured. With this method, the various lymphoid cells or combinations of them can be studied without the influence or interference of host's immune cells.

An extension of this method transfers cells from a mouse previously sensitized. These cells are injected into an x-irradiated, syngeneic host. Afterwards, the mice are challenged with antigen with hopes of eliciting a secondary response. B or T cells can be manipulated before transfer, and the influence of these cells in the x-irradiated mouse studied. A number of manipulations can be made from populations taken from a variety of places. The technique of transferring previously sensitized cells has become known as **adoptive transfer.**

This exercise uses the experiment described to show that cells involved in production of antibody to SRBC come from at least two sources, the thymus and spleen. The results also indicates that two **lymphoid cell populations cooperate** to produce antibody. The experiment shows that neither thymus cells nor spleen cells alone cause as great an immune response as does a combination of the two.

## MATERIALS

(Per pair or group of 4 students)

5 mice (4- to 6-week-old CBA)

Hanks' balanced salt solution (HBSS)

Glassware for buffer preparation

Filter sterilization apparatus

10% sheep red blood cell (SRBC) suspension

X-irradiation source

Surgical instruments (scissors, scalpel, forceps)

Unopette® white cell pipette and white blood cell diluting fluid

Hemacytometer

Ice

13 × 100-mm tubes

$CO_2$ for mouse euthanasia

Masking tape

70% ethyl alcohol

Small Petri dishes

Sterile rubber policeman

Capillary pipettes

Pipettes (1- and 5-ml)

Tubes for dilution series

18-gauge needle and 3-ml syringes

Centrifuge tubes

Heparin

Tuberculin needle and syringe

Mouse holder

Materials from exercise 22 (hemolytic plaque assay)

**119**

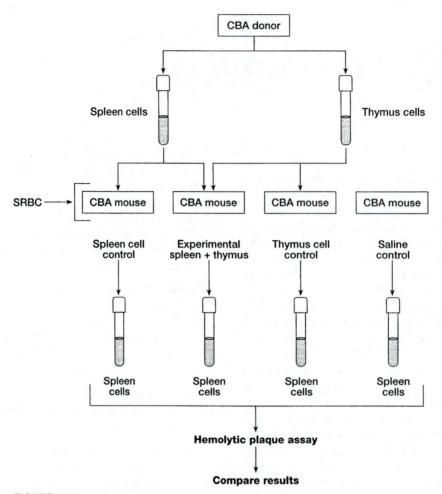

**FIGURE 24.1**
The experimental strategy for the reconstitution of the immune systems of irradiated mice with various populations of lymphocytes.

## PROCEDURE

1. Each pair of students will need five mice. Three mice will be reconstituted with: (1) thymus or (2) spleen cells or (3) a combination of these; one will serve as the **control** and the other will be the **spleen** and **thymus cell donor.** See figure 24.1 for the experimental design.

2. Use inbred 4- to 6-week-old CBA mice. This strain is chosen because lymphocytes from them are susceptible to 600–800 r. The instructor should determine this empirically before attempting this experiment since x-ray sensitivity may vary from laboratory to laboratory. CBA mice will serve both as donors and recipients of cells.

3. Prepare Hanks' balanced salt solution (HBSS) for use in making cell suspensions. The appendix discusses this preparation.

4. Prepare a 10% washed SRBC suspension; store it at 4° C until needed.

5. The instructor may have to consult with a radiologist or local hospital for the use of an x-ray machine. Irradiate mice individually in a plexiglass box and then given injections of donor spleen and thymus cells one day after irradiation. The dose should be produced with a potential of approximately 250 kV and 15 mA current to provide 600–800 r. After irradiation, keep the mice in **clean quarters** to minimize death due to infectious disease. Student pairs or groups will need 4 irradiated mice.

6. Prepare **spleen cells** that will be used to reconstitute the irradiated mice according to the outline in exercise 15. However, instead of RPMI 1640, use HBSS. After the last centrifugation step, dilute the cells to $5 \times 10^6$ cells/ml in HBSS containing 25 units heparin/ml. Store on ice until ready to use.

7. For preparation of **thymus cells,** kill a 4-week-old mouse in $CO_2$ or use cervical dislocation.

Tape the mouse to a surgical table with masking tape. Leave the abdominal and chest wall exposed. Swab these areas with 70% ethanol.

8. Refer to figure 15.2. Make an incision to expose the thoracic cage. The incision should extend from the submandibular region to the xyphoid process. Pull the skin away. Make an incision into the thoracic area with a scalpel and cut through the bone structure with scissors and separate the chest. Then cut through the mediastinal-pleural covering. The two thymic lobes should be visible, located just beneath the sternum in the upper portion of the mediastinum, the area just between the lungs.

9. Surgically remove the thymic lobes and place them in a small Petri dish containing HBSS. Tease the organ apart and use a sterile rubber policeman to produce a single-cell suspension of thymus cells. Alternatively, use a fine stainless steel sieve and force thymus fragments through it. With either method, larger clumps can be broken apart by aspiration through an 18-gauge needle, but remember that cells can be damaged if the aspiration procedure is not done carefully.

10. Let the remaining clumps settle, and aspirate the single cells in suspension with a capillary pipette. Pipette into a centrifuge tube and centrifuge at $650 \times g$ for 5 min. Add fresh HBSS, count the cells with a hemacytometer and dilute to $2.5 \times 10^8$ cells/ml in HBSS that contains 25 units heparin/ml. Store on ice until ready to use.

11. For intravenous injection, the student must use a mouse holder that immobilizes the mouse but yet allows injection into the tail. The mouse holder may be especially designed (figure 24.2) or may simply be a large (50 ml) plastic test tube or centrifuge tube fitted with a rubber stopper. Cut a notch in the stopper so that when the mouse is placed in the tube, the stopper can be put in place with the mouse's tail running along the notch in the stopper and outside the tube. Provide air vents.

12. Exercise 1 explained intravenous injection. Follow those directions to inject the lateral tail vein (on either side of the tail) of the irradiated mice.

13. Use the **experimental design** provided in figure 24.1 to inject mice with various cells. Slowly inject 0.2 ml of the spleen cell suspension from step 6 into two mice. Inject 0.2 ml of the thymus cell suspension from step 10 into a third mouse and into one of the mice injected with spleen cell suspension. This is the experimental mouse. Inject a fourth mouse with saline to serve as a control.

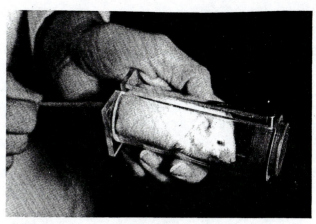

**FIGURE 24.2**
A mouse holder. Injection can be made into the tail with the mouse firmly held in this holder. There is little chance that the technician will harm the mouse or that the mouse will harm the technician.

14. Return the mice to clean quarters for 24 hr.
15. At the end of 24 hr, slowly inject 0.2 ml of the 10% SRBC suspension prepared in step 4 into each mouse.
16. Again return the mice to clean living quarters and leave for 5 days.
17. At the end of 5 days, kill them in $CO_2$ and perform the hemolytic plaque assay as described in exercise 22. Be sure to be **quantitative** for comparative purposes.

## DISCUSSION

Once a mouse receives more than 1,000 r, death may result for various reasons. For example, damage to the intestinal epithelium by higher doses can lead to death in less than 1 week. The dosage recommended in this exercise will selectively eliminate the radiosensitive lymphocytes without immediately affecting other cells.

This procedure as written should give a sufficient number of spleen and thymus cells for injection. It may be necessary, however, due to the inability of students to do a total thymectomy the first try, to use thymus cells collected from two mice. Experience has shown that, with careful surgical technique, $2.5 \times 10^8$ thymus cells can be obtained from a 4-week-old mouse.

## SELECTED REFERENCES

Claman, H. N., E. A. Chaperon, and R. F. Triplett. 1966. Thymus-marrow cell combinations: Synergism in antibody production. *Soc. Exp. Biol. Med.* 122:1167.

Mitchell, G. F., and J.F. A. P. Miller. 1968. Cell-to-cell interaction in the immune response. II. The source of hemolysin-forming cells in irradiated mice given bone marrow and thymus or thoracic duct lymphocytes. *J. Exp. Med.* 128:821.

Storer, J. B. 1966. Acute responses to ionizing radiation. In *Biology of the laboratory mouse.* Edited by E. L. Green. New York, NY: McGraw-Hill.

Taliaferro, H., and G. Taliaferro. 1976. Methods and applications of radiation in immunological research. In *Methods in immunology and immunochemistry.* Vol. 5. Edited by C. A. Williams and M. W. Chase. New York, NY: Academic Press.

# Formulations and Methods

This appendix contains the formulations for solutions and media as well as specific methods required to complete the exercises presented in this manual. Substitutions for these formulations may be made, but only at the discretion of the instructor.

## Adhesive Agar

Dip immunoelectrophoresis slides into a hot agar composed of 0.1 g of purified agar and 0.05 ml of glycerine in 100 ml distilled water. Drain the excess from the slide and slant to air dry.

## Barbital Buffer (pH 8.6)

| Sodium barbital | Barbituric acid |
|---|---|
| 15.47 g | 2.71 g |

Dissolve the components in 500 ml of distilled water. Heat to facilitate solubility of the ingredients and use mechanical stirring. Add distilled water to 1 liter and adjust the pH to 8.6 with 1 N NaOH.

## Blocking Buffer (pH 7.5)

Tris (10 mM) - 0.224 g
NaCl (0.9%) - 1.8 g
BSA (5%) - 10 g
Make up to 200 ml and adjust the pH to 7.5

## Blood Agar

| | |
|---|---|
| Trypticase soy agar (TSA) powder | 40.0 g |
| Distilled water | 1.0 l |
| Defibrinated sheep blood | 50.0 ml |

Melt and sterilize 1 liter of trypticase soy agar in a large Erlenmeyer flask in an autoclave at 121° C for 15 min. Warm 50 ml of defibrinated sheep blood to 50° C. After cooling the sterilized TSA to 50° C, aseptically transfer the blood to the TSA with gentle rotation of the flask. Pour 15 ml aliquots of the blood agar into sterile Petri dishes and allow to solidify. If bubbles form on the surface, flame gently with a Bunsen burner. The final pH should be 7.3.

## Brain Heart Infusion Broth and Agar

| | |
|---|---|
| Infusion from calf brain | 200.0 ml |
| Infusion from beef heart | 250.0 ml |
| Peptone | 10.0 g |
| Dextrose | 2.0 g |
| Sodium chloride | 5.0 g |
| Disodium phosphate | 2.5 g |
| Agar | 1.0 g |

Make up the ingredients to 1 liter with distilled water in a large Erlenmeyer flask. Use heat to bring to a boil. Cap and sterilize in an autoclave at 121° C for 15 min. The same formulation without the agar produces brain heart infusion broth. It is suggested that this medium be purchased in a dehydrated (powdered) form. Follow manufacturer's directions for preparation.

## Cell Count Determination

Use the method below for calculating cells/ml from a hemacytometer count where X is the number of cells in 80 small squares:

$$\text{Cells/ml} = [([X] \times [\text{dilution}] \times [4{,}000])/80] \times 1{,}000$$

The explanation for this calculation follows: The counting chamber is essentially a box. The smallest boxes (squares) have a length of 1/20 mm on each side, and the depth of the counting chamber is 1/10 mm. By counting the cells in one small square, you have determined the number of cells in 1/4,000 $mm^3$. Multiply this value times 4000 to calculate the number of cells in one $mm^3$. Since you counted 80 small squares, not just one, use the formula above. The 1,000 factor converts cells per $mm^3$ to cells per ml. The student may want to simplify the formula by multiplying the number of cells counted in 80 small squares by 50,000. Explain.

To determine the number of white blood cells after dilution in a Unopette® or a white cell pipette and counting in a hemacytometer use the following: The large squares are 1 mm long on each side. Since the hemacytometer chamber is 1/10 mm deep, the volume of blood counted is 1/10 $mm^3$. Four squares were counted so the volume is 4/10 $mm^3$. The dilution factor was 0.5/10 or 1/20 and therefore, the count represents the number of cells in $1/50$ mm$^3$. By multiplying the cells counted in 4 squares by 50, the total number of cells per mm$^3$ is obtained.

## Cell Dilution

The following formula is useful for preparing exact quantities of specific dilutions of cells.

$$(X_1)(Y_1) = (X_2)(Y_2)$$

where:

$X_1$ = Volume (ml) of original cell suspension needed. This is the value to be determined.

$Y_1$ = Number of cells/ml in the original cell suspension.

$X_2$ = Volume (ml) of diluted cell suspension wanted.

$Y_2$ = Number of cells/ml wanted in the diluted suspension.

For example, assume that you have determined that the original cell suspension has $2.3 \times 10^6$ cells/ml. The procedure directs you to dilute to $3 \times 10^5$ cells/ml and to prepare 12 ml of cell suspension. Solve the equation for x:

$$(X) (2.3 \times 10^6 \text{ cells/ml})$$

$$= (12 \text{ ml}) (3 \times 10^5 \text{ cells/ml})$$

$$X = \frac{(12 \text{ ml}) (3 \times 10^5 \text{ cells/ml})}{2.3 \times 10^6 \text{ cells/ml}}$$

$$X = 1.57 \text{ ml}$$

You would add 1.57 ml of the original cell suspension to 10.43 ml of diluent to produce 12 ml of a cell suspension containing $3 \times 10^5$ cells/ml.

## Coating Buffer

> Stock A—Mix 10.6 g Na$_2$CO$_3$ (anhydrous) in 500 ml of distilled water
> Stock B—Mix 8.4 g NaHCO$_3$ in 500 ml of distilled water

Add 80 ml of Stock A and 170 ml of Stock B and make up to a total volume of 500 ml with distilled water. The final pH should be 9.6.

## Coomassie Blue stain (for SDS-PAGE)

0.1% Coomassie Blue R-250 in fixative which is 40% methyl alcohol and 10% acetic acid

## Coomassie Brilliant Blue Reagent (for Bradford protein determination)

> Coomassie Brilliant Blue G-250 - 100 mg
> Ethanol (95%) - 50 ml

> Phosphoric acid (85%) - 100 ml

Combine these materials in a 1-liter volumetric flask and add water to 1 liter. Filter and store at 4° C.

## Destain Solution (for SDS-PAGE)

> 40% methanol and 10% acetic acid

## Double Diffusion Agar

Prepare a 1% solution of a purified agar in distilled water. A 1:1,000 dilution of merthiolate can be added as a preservative. Dispense into appropriate dishes.

## Diluting (Blocking) Buffer

Add 0.25 g of Tween 20 to 1.25 g of bovine serum albumin (BSA) (0.25%). Add phosphate-buffered saline (PBS) to 500 ml.

## Eagle's Minimal Essential Medium

| | |
|---|---|
| Calcium chloride (anhydrous) | 200.0 mg/l |
| Potassium chloride | 400.0 |
| Magnesium sulfate ($\cdot$ 7H$_2$O) | 200.0 |
| Sodium chloride | 6800.0 |
| Sodium bicarbonate | 2200.0 |
| Sodium phosphate ($\cdot$ H$_2$O) | 140.0 |
| Glucose | 1000.0 |
| Phenol red | 10.0 |
| L-arginine | 17.4 |
| L-cystine | 12.0 |
| L-glutamine | 292.0 |
| L-histidine | 8.0 |
| L-isoleucine | 26.0 |
| L-leucine | 26.0 |
| L-lysine | 29.2 |
| L-methionine | 7.5 |
| L-phenylalanine | 16.5 |
| L-threonine | 24.0 |
| L-tryptophane | 4.0 |
| L-tyrosin | 18.0 |
| L-valine | 23.5 |
| Biotin | 1.0 |
| D-Ca pantothenate | 1.0 |
| Choline chloride | 1.0 |
| Folic acid | 1.0 |
| i-Inositol | 2.0 |
| Nicotinamide | 1.0 |
| Pyridoxal HCl | 1.0 |
| Riboflavin | 0.1 |
| Thiamine HCl | 1.0 |

A number of vendors offer this medium in a liquid or powdered form. Liquid is shipped sterile; powdered media is rehydrated and should then be filter-sterilized. Store refrigerated.

## Gel Preserving Solution (for SDS-PAGE)

> Glycerol - 25 ml
>
> Ethanol - 50 ml
>
> Make up to 500 ml with water

## Hanks' Balanced Salt Solution (HBSS)

| | |
|---|---|
| D-glucose | 1.0 g/l |
| Phenol red | 0.01 |
| Potassium phosphate ($KH_2PO_4$) | 0.06 |
| Sodium phosphate ($Na_2HOP_4 \cdot 7H_2O$) | 0.09 |
| Calcium chloride | 0.14 |
| Potassium chloride | 0.4 |
| Sodium chloride | 8.0 |
| Magnesium chloride ($\cdot 6H_2O$) | 0.1 |
| Magnesium sulfate ($\cdot 7H_2O$) | 0.1 |
| Sodium bicarbonate | 0.35 |

Prepare two stock solutions. The first (solution A) should be composed of the first 4 components listed above and the second (solution B) the next 5 components. Mix solution A and B. Next, add the sodium bicarbonate to the mixture. Make sure that all ingredients are in solution and then filter-sterilize. The pH should be approximately 7.4. This solution can be purchased from a number of vendors in a liquid or powdered form. The liquid form is shipped sterile; powdered medium is rehydrated and should then be filter-sterilized. Store refrigerated.

## Hepes-Buffered Balanced Salt Solution (HEPES-BSS)

Prepare 6 stock solutions as follows:

1. Phosphate buffer is made by dissolving 22.9 g $KH_2PO_4$ and 19.5 g $K_2HPO_4$ in 950 ml of distilled water. Use KOH to adjust the pH to 7.2. Make up to 1 liter.
2. HEPES buffer is prepared by adding 80 g of HEPES to 13.4 g of NaOH and 950 ml of distilled water. Adjust the pH to 7.2 with NaOH or HCl. Make up to 1 liter.
3. NaCl (9.83 g/l)
4. KCl (12.5 g/l)
5. $CaCl_2$ (12.45 g/l)
6. $MgSO_4 \cdot 7H_2O$ (41.3 g/l)

Prepare the HEPES-BSS by adding the above stock solutions in the following proportions:

> 10 ml of stock solution 1
>
> 30 ml of stock solution 2
>
> 605 ml of stock solution 3
>
> 20 ml of stock solution 4
>
> 15 ml of stock solution 5
>
> 5 ml of stock solution 6
>
> Filter-sterilize the mixture and refrigerate to store.

## Immunoelectrophoresis Agar

Add 1.5 g of purified agar to 100 ml of barbital buffer (pH 8.6) and heat to melt the agar. Use this agar to prepare immunoelectrophoresis slides. Merthiolate (1:10,000) may be added as a preservative.

## Ketamine-Xylazine Anesthesia

Add 1 g of ketamine to 10 ml of sterile, distilled water. Dissolve. Add 30 mg of xylazine and mix. This can be stored at room temperature. For mouse anesthesia, dilute this 1:10 and inject intraperitoneally. Inject 100 mg ketamine/kg mouse body weight. Assuming the mouse weighs 0.018 kg, inject 0.18 ml for anesthesia. The range of the ketamine-xylazine solution for injection may vary from approximately 50 to 150 mg ketamine/kg depending upon the mouse and the particular species. For rabbits prepare a solution of 200 mg/ml as a stock solution. Inject 0.15 ml/lb of body weight intramuscularly for anesthesia.

## Lowry Reagent

Make the Lowry reagent by first preparing the following three solutions:

1. Sodium tartrate ($Na_2C_4H_4O_6 \cdot 2H_2O$)    2.0 g
   Add distilled $H_2O$ to 100 ml
2. Cupric sulfate ($CuSO_4 \cdot 5H_2O$)    1.0 g
   Add distilled $H_2O$ to 100 ml
3. Sodium carbonate ($Na_2CO_3$)    20.0 g
   Add sodium hydroxide (NaOH), 0.1 N to 1 liter.

To prepare the Lowry reagent from the above solutions, add 0.5 ml of reagent 1 to an Erlenmeyer flask. Add 0.5 ml of reagent 2 and mix. Finally add 50.0 ml of reagent 3 and mix once again. Prepare fresh daily. These reagents, as well as the Folin-Ciocalteu phenol reagent, can be purchased from a number of vendors.

## Peroxidase Substrate-Buffer Solution

Prepare a solution of o-phenylenediamine dihydrochloride at a concentration of 0.4 mg/ml in 0.05 M phosphate-citrate buffer, pH 5.0. Prepare the buffer by adding 25.7 ml of 0.2 M dibasic sodium phosphate (2.83 g in 100 ml distilled water) and 24.3 ml of 0.1 M citric acid (1.92 g in 100 ml distilled water) to 50 ml of distilled water. Adjust the pH to 5.0 if necessary. Important: Add 40 ml of 30% hydrogen peroxide per 100 ml of the substrate-buffer solution immediately prior to use.

## Phosphate Buffered Saline (PBS) (pH 7.2)

| | |
|---|---|
| NaCl | 8.77 g |
| $KH_2PO_4$ | 5.10 g |
| $Na_2HOP_4 \cdot 7H_2O$ | 10.50 g |

Make the solution up to 500 ml and determine that the pH is 7.2. Adjust if necessary. Add water to 1 liter. The final solution is 0.075 M. This makes a useful biological diluent for general purposes.

## Phosphate Buffered Saline (pH 5.3)

Prepare 500 ml of 0.1 M $Na_2PO_4$ and 500 ml of saline (8.5 g NaCl) and mix the two solutions. Adjust the pH to 5.3 with HCl.

## Ponceau S Stain

Prepare Ponceau S stain by adding 0.5 g of Ponceau S to 100 ml of 3% aqueous trichloroacetic acid.

## RPMI 1640

| | |
|---|---|
| $Ca(NO_3)_2 \cdot 4H_2O$ | 100.0 mg/l |
| KCl | 400.0 |
| $MgSO_4$ (anhydrous) | 48.9 |
| NaCl | 6000.0 |
| $Na_2HPO_4$ (anhydrous) | 800.0 |
| Glucose | 2000.0 |
| Glutathione (reduced) | 1.0 |
| Phenol red | 5.0 |
| L-arginine | 200.0 |
| L-asparagine (anhydrous) | 50.0 |
| L-aspartic acid | 20.0 |
| L-cystine · 2HCl | 65.2 |
| L-glutamic acid | 20.0 |
| L-glutamine | 300.0 |
| Glycine | 10.0 |
| L-histidine | 15.0 |
| Hydroxy-L-proline | 20.0 |
| L-isoleucine | 50.0 |
| L-leucine | 50.0 |
| L-lysine · HCl | 40.0 |
| L-methionine | 15.0 |
| L-phenylalanine | 15.0 |
| L-proline | 20.0 |
| L-serine | 30.0 |
| L-threonine | 20.0 |
| L-tryptophan | 5.0 |
| L-tyrosine | 20.0 |
| L-valine | 20.0 |
| p-aminobenzoic acid | 1.0 |
| d-biotin | 0.2 |
| D-Ca pantothenate | 0.3 |
| Choline chloride | 3.0 |
| Folic acid | 1.0 |
| i-Inositol | 35.0 |
| Nicotinamide | 1.0 |
| Pyridoxine · HCl | 1.0 |
| Riboflavin | 0.2 |
| Thiamine HCl | 1.0 |
| Vitamin $B_{12}$ | 0.005 |

A number of vendors offer this formulation in the liquid or powdered form. The liquid medium is shipped sterile; the powdered form is filter-sterilized after rehydration. Store refrigerated.

## Running (Electrode) Buffer pH 8.3 (5X stock)

Tris base - 9 g
Glycine - 43.2 g
Sodium dodecylsulfate (SDS) - 3 g

Make to 600 ml with distilled water. Store at 4° C and warm to 37° C before use if precipitation occurs. Dilute 60 ml of the 5X stock with 240 ml distilled water for a single electrophoretic run.

## Saline (and Ringer) Solution

Physiological saline, which is useful for the maintenance of microorganisms and mammalian cells, is a 0.85% solution of sodium chloride in water. Ringer solution is sometimes substituted for saline when diluting bacterial cells. The formulation for Ringer solution is:

| | |
|---|---|
| Sodium chloride | 2.15 g |
| Potassium chloride | 0.075 g |
| Calcium chloride (anhydrous) | 0.12 g |
| Sodium thiosulphate pentahydrate | 0.5 g |

Distilled water to 1 liter. Dilute this solution 1:4 before use; it will have a final pH of 6.6.

## Sample Buffer (SDS Reducing Buffer)

Distilled water - 4.0 ml

0.5 M Tris-HCl, pH 6.8 - 1.0 ml

Glycerol - 0.8 ml

10% (w/v) SDS - 1.6 ml

2-mercaptoethanol - 0.4 ml

0.05% (w/v) bromophenol blue - 0.2 ml

Store in a tightly capped bottle.

## Sodium Dodecyl Sulfate (SDS) (10%)

Add 10 ml SDS to 90 ml of distilled water. Store at room temperature.

## Top Agar (For Use in the Hemolytic Plaque Assay)

Add 0.7 g purified agar to 100 ml HEPES-BSS. Heat gently to melt the agar. Add 1 mg/ml DEAE-dextran, dispense into tubes and hold at 50° C.

## Transfer Buffer, pH 8.3

Tris (25 mM) - 3.03 g

Glycine (192 mM) - 14.4 g

Methanol (20% v/v) - 200 ml

Add distilled water to make 1 liter

Check the pH but do not adjust. Remake the solution if the pH is incorrect.

## Tris-HCl, 1.5 M, pH 8.8

Tris base - 27.23 g

Distilled water - 80 ml

Adjust the pH to 8.8 with 1 N HCl. Make up to 150 ml with distilled water and store at 4° C.

## Tris-HCl, 0.5 M, pH 6.8

Tris base - 6 g

Distilled water - 60 ml

Adjust the pH to 6.8 with 1 N HCl. Add distilled water to 100 ml and store at 4° C.

## Tris-Buffered Ammonium Chloride

Prepare a solution (solution A) containing 8.3 g/l $NH_4Cl$. Prepare a second solution (solution B) containing 20.6 g Tris base in 950 ml of water. Adjust the pH to 7.6 with HCl. Add water to make a total of 1 liter. Add 90 ml of solution A to 10 ml of solution B and mix. Bring the pH down to 7.2 with HCl.

## Trypan Blue Stain

Prepare the Trypan Blue stain by mixing 0.1% Trypan Blue in phosphate buffered saline (PBS), pH 7.3. Add an equal volume of the stain and the cells to be stained and gently mix. Prepare a wet mount and observe with light microscopy. Stained cells are considered to be nonviable.

## Tris-Buffered Saline

Tris (20 mM) - 2.422 g

NaCl - 29.255 g

Make up to 1 liter in distilled water

## Wash Buffer (for ELISA)

Add 0.25 g of Tween 20 (0.05%) to 500 ml of PBS.

## Wash Buffer (for Western Blots)

Tween 20 (0.3%) - 3 ml

Make up to 1 liter with Tris-buffered saline

## White Cell Diluting Fluid

This solution causes lysis of red blood cells without affecting the viability of the white blood cells. Using this procedure, the white cells become more visible microscopically. Prepare 0.5% acetic acid with a small amount of crystal violet.

## Wright's Stain

This preparation should yield sharp results.

1. Prepare a stock solution as follows:

| | |
|---|---|
| Wright stain (commercially available) | 1 g |
| Glycerol | 50 ml |
| Methanol (100%) | 50 ml |

Mix the glycerol and methanol and then add the stain. Store at room temperature.

2. Prepare a working solution as follows:

| | |
|---|---|
| Stock stain solution (from above) | 4 ml |
| Acetone | 3 ml |
| Phosphate buffer (15 M, pH 6.5) | 2 ml |
| Distilled water | 31 ml |

Mix together.

Immerse fixed blood smears in the working solution in a staining jar. Stain for 5 minutes. Wash gently in distilled water. Air dry and observe microscopically. The clearly visible structures will appear blue, red or purple.

# Vendors of Supplies and Equipment

The following list includes a number of suppliers of materials (biologicals, reagents, glassware, plasticware, etc.) and equipment used in the exercises presented in this manual. However, the list does not contain all possible sources for materials or equipment.

Aldrich Chemical Company
P.O. Box 2060
Milwaukee, WI 53201
(800) 558–9160

American Type Culture Collection
12301 Parklawn Drive
Rockville, MD 20852
(800) 638–6597

Amicon
72 Cherry Hill Drive
Beverly, MA 01915
(800) 343–1397

J. T. Baker
222 Red School Lane
Phillipsburg, NJ 08865
(800) 582–2537

Baxter Diagnostics, Inc. Division
Scientific Products
1430 Waukegan Road
McGraw Park, IL 60085
(800) 964–5227

Beckman Instruments
846 E. Algonquin Road
Schaumburg, IL 60173
(800) 742–2345

Becton Dickinson Labware
1 Becton Drive
Franklin Lakes, NJ 07417
(800) 235–5953

Behring Diagnostics, Inc.
151 University Avenue
Westwood, MA 02090
(800) 321–3394

Bio-Rad Laboratories
2000 Alfred Nobel Drive
Hercules, CA 94547
(800) 424–6723

Boehringer Mannheim Biochemicals
P.O. Box 50414
Indianapolis, IN 46250
(800) 262–1640

Burroughs Wellcome
3030 Cornwallis Road
Research Triangle Park, NC 27709
(800) 722–9292

Calbiochem
P.O. Box 12087
La Jolla, CA 92039
(800) 854–3417

Charles River Laboratories
251 Ballardvale Street
Wilmington, MA 01887
(800) 522–7287

Cole-Parmer
7425 North Oak Park Avenue
Niles, IL 60714
(800) 323–4340

Corning
Corning, NY 14831
(607) 974–9000

Corning Costar
1 Alewife Center
Cambridge, MA 02140
(800) 492–1110

Difco Laboratories
P.O. Box 331058
Detroit, MI 48232
(800) 521–0851

Du Pont NEN Research Products
549 Albany Street
Boston, MA 02118
(800) 551–2121

Dynatech Laboratories
14340 Sullyfield Circle
Chantilly, VA 22021
(800) 336–4543

EC Apparatus
3831 Tyrone Boulevard North
St. Petersburg, FL 33709
(800) 327–2643

Fisher Scientific
1241 Ambassador Road
ST. Louis, MO 63132
(800) 766–7000

FMC Bioproducts
191 Thomaston Street
Rockland, ME 04841
(800) 341–1574

Gelman Sciences
600 South Wagner Road
Ann Arbor, MI 48103
(800) 521–1520

Genzyme
1 Kendall Square
Cambridge, MA 02139
(800) 332–1042

GIBCO/BRL
P.O. Box 68
Grand Island, NY 14072
(800) 828–6686

Helena Laboratories
1530 Lindbergh Drive
P.O. Box 752
Beaumont, TX 77704
(800) 231–5663

Hoefer Scientific Instruments
P.O. Box 77387
San Francisco, CA 94107
(800) 227–4750

ICN Biomedicals
3300 Highland Avenue
Costa Mesa, CA 92626
(800) 854–0530

International Equipment Co.
300 Second Avenue
Needham Heights, MA 02194
(800) 843–1113

Isco, Inc.
P.O. Box 5347
Lincoln, NE 68505
(800) 228–4250

J. T. Baker
222 Red School Lane
Phillipsburg, NJ 08865
(800) 582–2537

Miles Laboratories
195 West Birch Street
Kankakee, IL 60901
(800) 227–9412

Millipore Corporation
397 Williams Street
Marlboro, MA 01752
(800) 645-5476

Murex Diagnostics
3075 Northwoods Circle
Norcross, GA 30071
(800) 334–8570

Nalge
Nalgene Labware
75 Panorama Creek Drive
Rochester, NY 14602
(716) 586–8800

Nunc
2000 North Aurora Road
Naperville, IL 60563
(800) 288–6862

Pharmacia Biotech and Pharmacia
Diagnostics
P.O. Box 1327
800 Centenial Avenue
Piscataway, NJ 08855
(800) 526–3593

Rainin Instrument Co.
Mack Road, Box 4026
Woburn, MA 01888
(800) 225–5392

Sartorius Corporation
131 Hartland Boulevard
Edgewood, NY 11717
(800) 368–7178

Sigma Chemical Co.
P.O. Box 14508
St. Louis, MO 63178
(800) 325–3010

Sorvall
31 Pecks Lane
Newtown, CT 06470
(800) 551–2121

Taconic Farms
273 Hover Avenue
Germantown, NY 12526
(518) 537–6208

Thomas Scientific
P.O. Box 99
99 High Hill Road
Swedesboro, NJ 08085
(800) 345–2100

VWR Scientific
P.O. Box 7900
San Francisco, CA 94120
(800) 932–5000

Worthington Biochemical
Halls Mill Road
Freehold, NJ 07728
(800) 445–9603

# Index

Acid fuchsin, 106
Acrylamide, 64
Adherence, 24
Adhesive agar, 106
Adoptive transfer, 119
Affinity chromatography, 59, 101
Agar, 49
Agarose, 59, 101
Agglutination, 11, 35, 36, 39, 42, 43, 44
Agglutination, bacterial, 37
Agglutination, passive, 35
Agglutination test, 38
Albumin, 16
Allergen, 113
Allergy, 18, 113
Alloantigen, 89
Allogenic recipient, 115
Allograft (homograft), 115, 118
Alpha-1-antitrypsin, 22
Alpha-2-macroglobulin, 22
Alpha-fetoprotein, 49
Ammonium sulfate precipitation, 104
Anaphylactic sensitivity, 113
Anaphylactic shock, 114, 115
Anaphylaxis, 8, 113
Anesthesia, 7, 8
Animal, experimental, 6, 8
Anti-A isoantibody, 36
Anti-B isoantibody, 36
Antibody, 4, 8, 11, 16, 35, 39, 40, 45, 49, 109
Antibody, agglutinating, 35, 37
Antibody excess, 29
Antibody, fluorescent, 76
Antibody, homologous, 29
Antibody production, 4
Antibody titer, 30
Antibody-dependent cytotoxic
    hypersensitivity, 113
Antibody-enzyme conjugate, 55
Anti-BSA, 29, 30, 50, 51, 115
Anticoagulant, 8, 16
Antigen, 29, 35, 39, 40, 41, 45, 49
Antigen excess, 29, 31, 49
Antigen, particulate, 35
Antigen, soluble, 35
Antigen, surface, 85
Antigenic determinant, 4, 5
Antigen-presenting cell, 89
Anti-HCG, 40
Antimicrobial, 21
Antinuclear antibody, 41, 42
Antiserum, 30
Antistreptolysin O (ASO) test, 42
Arteritis, 114
Aseptic technique, 4, 9, 78, 79
Autopipette, 12
Autoradiography, 109

B cell, 81, 89, 93, 119
*Bacillus cereus,* 23
Bacterin, 4
Basophil, 18
Benzidine dihydrochloride, 111
Betadine, 116
Betalysin, 22
Bio-Ice cooling unit, 71
Biotin-avidin-enzyme conjugate, 44
Bis-acrylamide, 64
Blastogenic response, 89, 91
Bleb 7, 116
Blood, 15, 16
Blood group (ABO), 36, 37
Blood transfusion, 36
Blue Dextran, 103
Bone marrow, 16, 81, 119
Bovine serum albumin (BSA), 29, 33, 50,
    51, 116
Bradford method, 33
Brain heart infusion agar, 4, 23
Brain heart infusion broth, 4, 6
Buffer, 48, 49
Buffer, barbital, 50, 106, 107
Buffer, binding, 60
Buffer, blocking, 56, 72
Buffer, coating, 56, 61
Buffer, diluting, 56
Buffer, elution, 60
Buffer, regeneration, 61
Buffer, running, 68, 70
Buffer, transfer, 71, 72
Buffer, wash, 56, 61, 72

Capping, 82, 84
Carbon dioxide asphyxiation, 24
Cardiac puncture, 7, 8, 9
Carrier, 35, 39
Cell, blood, 16
Cell culture, 77
Cell harvester, 91
Cell life cycle, 4
Cell, stem, 16
Cell-mediated hypersensitivity, 114
Cell-mediated hypersensitivity reaction, 113
Cell-mediated immune response, 85
Cellulose acetate paper, 45, 47, 48
Centers for Disease Control and Prevention, 19
Centricon microconcentrators, 104
Centrifugation, 15
Chromatography, 101
Chromogen, 55
Clot, 8, 16
Clotting factors, 16
Colony forming units, 23, 24
Column chromatography, 101, 102

Complement, 21, 49 109, 111, 113
Complex-mediated hypersensitivity reaction,
    113
Concanavalin A (ConA), 76, 89, 91, 93
Contamination, 5
Continuous cell line, 77
Control, 13, 37, 38, 39, 44, 71, 84, 96, 116,
    117, 120
Control, antigen, 38
Coomassie Blue, 63
Coomassie Brilliant Blue, 33, 34
Coulter STKS, 18
C-reactive protein, 22, 49
C-reactive protein (CRP) test, 42
Criss-cross serial dilution analysis, 55
Culture, 76
Culture medium, 77
Cytokine, 93
Cytolysis, 21
Cytotoxic, 85

D10.G4.1 cell, 97
DEAE-dextran, 110
Delayed hypersensitivity reaction, 113
Density centrifugation, 85
Deoxyribonucleohistone (DNP), 41
Destain solution, 70
Detergent, 13
Dextran sulfate, 79
Dialysis, 101, 102
Dialysis tubing, 102
Diluent, 11
Dilution, 11
Dilution, ten-fold, 11
Dilution, two-fold, 12
Diploid cell strain, 77
Disease, 18
Disease, infectious, 21
DNA synthesis, 89
Double diffusion, 49
Double gel diffusion, 105
Dye, tracing, 45

E receptor, 86
Eagles minimal essential medium (EMEM), 24
Effector cell, 89
Egg albumin, 6
Electrophoresis, 45, 63, 71, 105
ELISA, direct, 55
ELISA, indirect, 55
Endoreticular system, 22, 23
Endotoxin, 9
Endpoint reaction, 11
Enzyme, 41
Enzyme-Linked Immunosorbent Assay
    (ELISA), 55